Neuroscience and Art

A Collection of Essays

Neuroscience and Art

A Collection of Essays

Ambar Chakravarty
MD FRCPC FRCP FRCPE FIAN
Honorary Professor and Emeritus Consultant
Department of Neurology
Vivekananda Institute of Medical Science
Kolkata, West Bengal, India
Past-President, Indian Academy of Neurology (2005–2006)

JAYPEE
JAYPEE BROTHERS MEDICAL PUBLISHERS
The Health Sciences Publisher
New Delhi | London

JAYPEE **Jaypee Brothers Medical Publishers (P) Ltd**

Headquarters
EMCA House
23/23-B, Ansari Road, Daryaganj
New Delhi 110 002, India
Landline: +91-11-23272143, +91-11-23272703
+91-11-23282021, +91-11-23245672
E-mail: jaypee@jaypeebrothers.com

Corporate Office
Jaypee Brothers Medical Publishers (P) Ltd.
4838/24, Ansari Road, Daryaganj
New Delhi 110 002, India
Phone: +91-11-43574357
Fax: +91-11-43574314
E-mail: jaypee@jaypeebrothers.com

Overseas Office
JP Medical Ltd.
83, Victoria Street, London
SW1H 0HW (UK)
Phone: +44-20 3170 8910
Fax: +44(0)20 3008 6180
E-mail: info@jpmedpub.com

Website: www.jaypeebrothers.com
Website: www.jaypeedigital.com

Inquiries for bulk sales may be solicited at: jaypee@jaypeebrothers.com

Neuroscience and Art: A Collection of Essays / ***Ambar Chakravarty***

First Edition: **2025**

Reprint: **2025**

ISBN: 978-93-6616-714-5

Printed in India

Remembrance

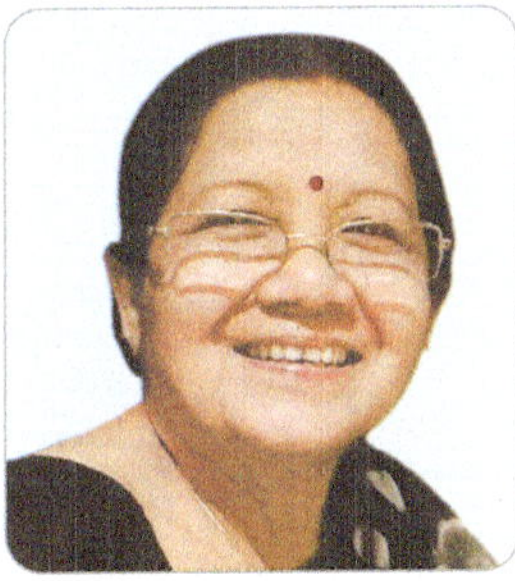

Srilekha

(1948–2024)

My wife of 50 years and a longtime companion in my journey in the World of Arts

Dedication

Anuradha

"A Friend in Need is a Friend Indeed"

PREFACE

When I was a young child, my father taught me, "If you want to learn English, speak in English, read in English, write in English, think in English, and dream in English". Later, while doing my residency, I learnt that the same principles apply to learning neurology as well. It had been the thinking and dreaming in neurosciences which stimulated me to enter the world of arts and its relationship to neurosciences and finally the publication of this collection of essays.

Questions would arise: What is art and what is the relationship between art and neuroscience? Semir Zeki, a contemporary celebrated neurophysiologist and a great scholar in various aspects of art, wrote in 1999, "An artist is a Neurologist"; the contents of this book would support Zeki's contention to a great extent.

Like speech, art, especially visual art, may be defined as a symbolic expression of one's own thought. The artist expresses his/her experience, idea, thought, and/or opinion on a subject crossing his/her mind or visually or auditorily perceived. Art is an expression of human creativity that is not observed in any other living creature. It is indeed not a very commonly encountered skill and can only be learned by extensive study, practice, and observation. Through art, it is possible not only to record or describe objects, events, and moments, but also to express feelings, opinions, and attitudes. Modern neuroscience has the privilege to investigate the processes of artistic performance in a healthy brain by means of advanced neuroimaging techniques such as functional neuroimaging.

Until recent times, neuroscientists could only speculate which brain functions are involved in artistic processes by observing works of neurological patients who possessed artistic talents. The right hemisphere mostly controls metaphoric thinking, solution finding, and synthesizing. It is the center of visualization, imagination, and conceptualization, all components of artistic production. However, the left hemisphere is still needed for artistic work to achieve balance by partly suppressing excessive creative output of the right hemisphere and for the execution part of a creative process, namely drawing, painting, dancing, and instrumental handling. A very specific functional organization of brain areas is involved in visual art production and appreciation. Different parts of visual cortex are activated, depending on the type of picture viewed (colors, objects, faces, position of objects in space, motion or static pictures).

This book would be a unique one where the close relationship between visual artistic production and appreciation is discussed in detail as well as how this intricate relationship gets disturbed in different diseases of the central nervous system. The book includes 14 chapters, all written by the author, some of which had earlier been published in national and international journals and would be reproduced with modifications, and some of the topics had been talked about by the author as guest lectures and orations. Nearly half of the topics concentrate on the basic scientific aspects of how art is produced and what techniques artists employ to increase the aesthetic value of their art works without having a clear idea about the brain areas, the stimulation of which gives rise to the "Ah!" expression in the mind of the viewer. Artists most likely do this by following certain fundamental principles of art making which are based on the fundamental principles of brain functioning. Contrary to the commonly used statement "*Beauty lies in the eyes of the beholder*", modern neuroscience and neuroimaging have clearly established that "*Beauty lies in the brain of the beholder*". The rest of the essays discuss how visual artworks get affected when artists are ill with different diseased conditions affecting the brain which often help us to understand the functions of those areas of the brain in healthy individuals.

This book is not made solely for neurologists but for all categories of physicians (and nonmedical personnel too) who have interests outside their chosen specialty and have reasonable knowledge about the structure and functions of different brain regions. To the best of my knowledge, no such book had yet been published from any Asian country and only a very few exist in the western world. The subject of Neuroscience and Art on the whole rests on isolated case reports and some detailed review articles needing profound knowledge of neuropsychology for their full appreciation. This book would hopefully stimulate interests among physicians on the neuroscientific basis of art and creativity in relatively simple language. Fine art has at least three subdivisions, namely Visual Art, Music, and Literature. Visual Arts and Literature have been discussed in fair detail in this book, but no discussions have been made on the neuroscientific basis of music, principally because I do not consider myself to be competent enough to write about the fundamentals of musicology and its neural basis, although I remain an ardent music lover. Some of the illustrations used had been from my personal collections, some had been photographed from temples, caves, museums, and art galleries, and a few reproduced from published works with permissions.

My journey into the world of arts began some 20 years back in close companionship with my wife Srilekha and together we studied arts, visited numerous galleries and museums around the world, and made our residence a mini art museum. The idea of producing such a book had been in our minds for the past 3 years or so. Her rather sudden and untimely passing away early this year made myself feel like a pilotless ship in a vast ocean and I had difficulty in putting myself back in my long chosen path of pursuing profession and academics simultaneously. This book is primarily written as a mark of remembrance to a great person who sacrificed a lot as the *Front Engine* in my life's journey for the past 50 years.

Anuradha had been a patient of mine for the past 27 years fighting with multiple sclerosis. She later became a close family friend, specially with my wife. She really behaved like a true friend during the darkest days of my life, arguing with me, ordering me, and giving me all sorts of encouragement. The result had been the production of two books, the present one and an earlier one which is currently in press. I am much indebted to her and dedicate this book to her ... my very efficient *Back Engine*.

Ambar Chakravarty

Ratha Yatra 2024

CONTENTS

CHAPTER

1

What is Art? What is Beauty? Neuropsychological and Philosophical Perspectives

INTRODUCTION

Like speech, art, especially visual art, may be defined as a symbolic expression of one's own thought. The artist expresses his/her experience, idea, thought and/or opinion on a subject crossing his/her mind or visually or auditorily perceived. Art is an expression of human creativity that is not observed in any other living creature. It is indeed not a very commonly encountered skill which can only be learned by extensive study, practice, and meticulous observation. A good piece of art not only records or describe objects, events, and moments, but also can express feelings, opinions, and attitudes. Paul Klee, the Swiss painter said: "Art does not reproduce the visible; rather it makes the invisible, visible."[1] Today, we have the privilege to investigate the processes of artistic performance in a healthy brain by means of advanced neuroimaging techniques like functional neuroimaging [functional magnetic resonance imaging (fMRI)].

Until some years back, neuroscientists could only speculate what brain functions are involved in artistic processes by observing art works created by patients with various localizable neurological disorders who possessed artistic talents. Interestingly, in relation to cerebral hemispheric dominance, less creative people have marked hemispheric dominance and more creative people have less marked hemispheric dominance.[2,3] The right hemisphere mostly controls metaphoric thinking, solution finding, and synthesizing. It is the center of visualization, imagination, and conceptualization, all of which are needed for visual artistic production. However, the left hemisphere is still needed for artistic work to achieve balance by partly suppressing excessive creative output of the right hemisphere and for the executive part of a creative process, namely drawing, painting, dancing, and instrumental handling.[4] A very specific functional organization of brain areas is involved in visual art production and appreciation as would be discussed elsewhere in this volume. Different parts of visual cortex are activated, depending on the type of picture viewed (colors, objects, faces, position of objects in space, motion, or static pictures).[5-7] Both right and left hemispheres of the brain are involved in the process of complete musical experience. The frontal cortex has a significant role in rhythm and melody perception. The centers for perceiving pitch and certain aspects of melody and harmony and rhythm are identified in the right hemisphere (amelodia and aprosodia are seen in right hemispheric diseases). Left hemisphere is important for processing rapid changes in frequency and intensity of tune. Several cortical areas are activated during listening to music which can explain the impact of listening to music on emotions, cognition, and motor performances.[8-10]

WHAT IS BEAUTY?

Beauty is just one of many undefined esthetic experiences.[11,12] Most philosophers (like Plato, Aristotle, Kant, and Hegel) state that experiencing beauty involves the experience of pleasure. Philosophers like Plato and Kant observe that one's own beauty experiences seem universally valid. Hume and Santayana, in contrast, do not claim that beauty is necessarily perceived as universal. A further dimension that differentiates philosophers' conceptions of beauty is surprise. Hegel and Aristotle viewed surprise as a central element of experiencing beauty, whereas it played little role for others (like Kant, Plato, and Hume). Some (like Santayana) even went so far as to claim that surprise is a measure of ugliness, and thus detrimental to beauty.

Why it is that a large number of people find a particular piece of art, music, dance, or a poem beautiful (e.g., da Vinci's paintings or Tagore's poetry). Does "*beauty lies in the eye of the beholder*"? Zeki and his colleagues conducted a study the results of which have revealed that a beauty experience is indeed in the beholder, though not in the eye, but in the brain. They studied 21 subjects in whom brain fMRI scanning was performed during looking at something beautiful or listening to something that the subject liked. They showed that during these actions, activation of medial orbitofrontal cortex occurred and it is assumed that also other stimuli that person finds beautiful would activate the same area.[13]

Zeki pointed out in his book, "Vision of the Brain", that all human experience is mediated through the brain and is not solely the product of the outside world. He writes "The more important the experience, the more it can reveal about the fundamental properties of the brain."[14]

Esthetics is a very important part of human life like love and hate. Although we may rarely be conscious of it, esthetic experience gives value to everything we are, all we experience, and everything we do. Theoretically without it, life would be a shapeless, meaningless, and colorless series of sensations, events, and reactions. Esthetic experience achieves its most refined form in the fine arts like visual arts and music.

HOW DOES BEAUTY FEEL?

Emotions accompany and form a substantial part of our experiences of art and other related creative endeavors and hence affective responses play a central role in processing of visual and other forms of art. Unfortunately, there is hardly any standardized classification of and measurement tool for such emotions. Such emotions arise when a person perceives and evaluates a stimulus (e.g., an object of art) for its esthetic appeal or virtues. The concept of esthetic emotion—like the more general concept of emotion—is prototypically organized and lacks sharp boundaries.

MUSIC AND BRAIN: A BRIEF NOTE

The connection between music and brain functioning is known for centuries. In an ancient (>3,000 years) Chinese book, "The Book of Changes/Wisdom", it is written: "Music has the power to ease the tension within the heart and to lessen and loosen obscure emotions." Pythagoras, in the 6th century, noted that fine pleasant tunes represented particular mathematical relations or harmony and he supported using this harmonic music in an attempt to achieve harmony of bodily functions. His students prescribed specific tunes and dances as a cure for mood disorders.[15]

Music has stimulatory actions on specific regions of the brain and it affects processes responsible for memory, motor control, timing, and language. fMRI studies have shown reorganization of motor and auditory cortex in professional musicians probably related to changes in degree in connectivity. Furthermore, other studies have analyzed the changes in neurotransmitter and serum hormone levels in correlation to music. Music, thus, is biologically a part of human life and not just esthetically related.

Ramon Cajal wrote:[16] "Every man can, if he so desires, become a sculptor of his own brain." Current interest in brain plasticity-related experiments has shown that brain is capable of making new connections, activating new pathways, and unmasking secondary roads. Music is one of the most frequently investigated tool/stimulus for neuroplasticity. Studies have shown that the exposure of pregnant women and neonates to music promotes the development of the brain and the inner ear of child. Thus, exposure to music in early life reorganizes the brain connections with consequently improved coordination and other motor skills. Music can also induce neuroplastic changes in adult brains, both normal and injured, which includes alteration of the auditory cortex after attentive listening to music regularly for a prolonged period. The Mozart effect refers to the enhancement of performance or changing of neuropsychological activity after regular listening to Mozart's music.

The basis of the Mozart effect lies at the neuroplastic reorganization of the cerebral cortex that may resonate with the captivating qualities of Mozart's music.[17] "Brain music" refers to the use of frequency, amplitude, and duration of musical sound similar to Chopin music which is able to move the brain from an anxious state to a more relaxed state and has positive effect on insomnia and fatigue.

The use of music as a therapy showed its success in depressive patients after stroke.[18] The rehabilitation of stroke patients can be improved by incorporation of music listening in the therapy. Music listening increases blood flow in patients suffering from acute ischemic stroke and, therefore, enhances the post-stroke recovery.[19] Music is beneficial if created as well.

Singing may induce changes of physiologic markers of happiness; the serotonin, norepinephrine, and β-endorphin levels were significantly higher after than before singing and stress hormone epinephrine was reduced by singing.[20]

Artistic training, especially in art interested persons, may also improve attention and cognition. The likely reason is activity-dependent neuroplasticity; the focused training in any of the arts activates attention networks that are needed in learning and memory processes.

Music has a beneficiary effect on brain plasticity, music training in children for a number of years revealed significantly better results on general measures of intelligence, in reading fluency and in performance in the geometry skills compared to results of children who did not receive such training.[21,22]

CONCLUDING REMARKS

In summary, art relates to human creativity; it is a skill that can be learned by thorough study, practice, and keen observation. Brain is capable of making new connections and activating new pathways; it is "plastic" in nature. Music is a strong stimulus for neuroplasticity which can be utilized in therapy of patients with mood and cognitive impairments especially following strokes. In the field of visual art, brain lesion can lead to neurological lesions leading to significant impairment of artistic work. Lesions affecting the left deficits hemisphere may reveal new artistic dimensions, disinhibiting the right hemisphere where work is more spontaneous and emotional with the gain of artistic quality, often leading to de novo development of such qualities, a phenomenon called "paradoxical functional facilitation".

REFERENCES

1. Giedion-Welcker C. Klee. Hamburg: Rowohlt; 1998.
2. Katz AN. Creativity and the right cerebral hemisphere: towards a physiologically based theory of creativity. J Creat Behav. 1978;12:253-64.
3. York GK. The cerebral localization of creativity. In: Rose FC (Ed). Neurology of the Arts: Paintings, Music, Literature. London: Imperial College Press; 2004. pp. 1-9.
4. Hoppe KD. Hemispheric specialization and creativity. Psychiatr Clin N Am. 1988;11:303-15.
5. Zeki S, Watson JD, Lueck CJ, Friston KJ, Kennard C, Frackowiak RS. A direct demonstration of functional specialization in human visual cortex. J Neurosci. 1991;11:641-9.
6. Zeki S, Marini L. Three cortical stages of colour processing in the human brain. Brain. 1998;121:1669-85.
7. Zeki S. Neural Concept Formation and Art: Dante, Michaelangelo, Wagner. In: Rose FC (Ed). Neurology of the Arts: Paintings, Music, Literature. London: Imperial College Press; 2004. pp. 13-41.
8. Tramo MJ. Biology and music. Music of the hemispheres. Science. 2001;291:54-6.
9. Tramo MJ, Shah GD, Braida LD. Functional role of auditory cortex in frequency processing and pitch perception. J Neurophysiol. 2002;87:122-39.
10. Janata P, Grafton ST. Swinging in the brain: shared neural substrates for behaviors related to sequencing and music. Nat Neurosci. 2003;6:682-7.
11. Leder H, Nadal M. Ten years of a model of aesthetic appreciation and aesthetic judgments: The aesthetic episode - Developments and challenges in empirical aesthetics. Br J Psychol. 2014;105(4):443-64.

12. Pelowski M, Markey PS, Forster M, Gerger G, Leder H. Top-down and bottom-up: Front to back: Comment on "Move me, astonish me... delight my eyes and brain: The Vienna Integrated Model of top-down and bottom-up processes in Art Perception (VIMAP) and corresponding affective, evaluative, and neurophysiological correlates". Phys Life Rev. 2017;21:148-9.
13. Ishizu T, Zeki S. A neurobiological enquiry into the origins of our experience of the sublime and beautiful. Front Hum Neurosci. 2014;8:891.
14. Zeki S. A Vision of the Brain. Oxford: Blackwell Scientific Publications; 1993.
15. Karamanides D. Pythagoras: Pioneering mathematician and musical theorist of ancient Greece. New York: Rosen Publishing, Inc.; 2006.
16. Cajal SR. Histologie du systeme nerveux de l'homme & des vertebres. Instituto Ramon y Cajal: Consejo Superior de Investigaciones Cientificas; 1955.
17. Campbell D. The Mozart Effect. New York: Harper Collins; 2009.
18. Särkämö T, Tervaniemi M, Laitinen S, Forsblom A, Soinila S, Mikkonen M, et al. Music listening enhances cognitive recovery and mood after middle cerebral artery stroke. Brain. 2008;131:866-76.
19. Antić S, Jensen U, Lovrenčić Huzjan A, Vuković V, Mukhtarova R, Ferreira Sao Silva Santos SV, et al. Changes of cerebral hemodynamics during music perception: a functional transcranial Doppler study. Acta Clin Croat. 2006;45:301-7.
20. Biegl T. Glücklich singen – singend glücklich? Gesang als Beitrag zum Wohlbefinden. Serotonin, Noradrenalin, Adrenalin, Dopamin und Beta-Endorphin als psychophysiologische Indikatoren. Wien: Diplomarbeit; 2004.
21. Hyde KL, Lerch J, Norton A, Forgeard M, Winner E, Evans AC, et al. Musical training shapes structural brain development. J Neurosci. 2009;29:3019-25.
22. Posner MI, Patoine B. (2009). How arts training improves attention and cognition. [online] Available from https://www.researchgate.net/publication/255655328_How_Arts_Training_Improves_Attention_and_Cognition. [Last accessed January, 2025]

CHAPTER 2

The Creative Brain

INTRODUCTION

"You see things; and you say 'why' but I dream things that never were; and I say 'why not'."

—George Bernard Shaw

These few lines of George Bernard Shaw beautifully illustrate the basic concept of creativity which essentially is an abstract phenomenon. It is a complex neuro-psycho-philosophical concept which is difficult to define literally. Creativity can be defined as a mental and social process involving the generation of new ideas or concepts, or new association of the creative mind between existing ideas and concepts. Creativity is fueled by the process of either conscious or unconscious insight. An alternative conception of creativeness is that it is simply the act of making something new (*http://www.wikipedia.com*). Recently, Meyers and Gerstman[1] compiled the "unconventional wisdom from 20 accomplished minds" in their book, "Creativity". Here, while a famous American playwright (Edward Albee) comments that "the only thing that separates the creative from the noncreative is the fact that creative people are not content merely to have the experience, but insist on commenting on it"; one famous architect (Daniel Libeskind) writes "I think creativity is something eternal, because it is an encounter with a moment of time—creativity is not only the search for the new, it can be a rediscovery on the newness of thousands of years ago, which is still unsurpassed in some way"; according to a famous author (Erica Jong), "creativity is mysterious... a creative person is someone who sees the world differently, and does not accept that structures that most people unthinkingly accept"; a musician feels "you cannot quite write directions on how to be creative—it is something that just happens because that is what creative people are all about"; and lastly a contemporary artist of much fame (Chuck Close) feels "...The most exciting thing in the visual arts is to see something that actually does not look like art". So you see the divergent views about creativity even among creative people. The reason probably is that creativity (like intelligence) is often domain specific.

The present author particularly likes the concept proposed by Bronowski.[2] Creativity is finding unity in what appears to be diversity. Great art works have a myriad of colors and forms and great musical works have a large variety of melodies and rhythms, but in both paintings and symphonies, the artist is able to develop a thread that unites diverse elements and displays order. Creative scientist such as Copernicus was able to see order in what appeared to be a disorderly solar system and Einstein was able to see the thread that unites matter and energy. Establishing the root of this novel orderly relationship through the eyes of a neuroscientist would be the prime objective of this chapter. In doing so, the author would first make a critical review of proposed concepts of creative cognition, suggest some new ones which the author would try to prove to be essential in the genesis of the cognitive process and would then try to hypothesize on an all embracing conceptual construct for creative cognition and output.

CREATIVITY THEORY

Years ago, Graham Wallas[3] suggested that creativity has four stages—preparation, incubation, illumination, and verification. Preparation is the acquisition of the skills and knowledge that allow a person to create. Einstein developed superb skills in physics and mathematics before he made his discoveries and Pablo Picasso learned to draw forms and mix colors (first from his father and then at art schools in La Coruna, Barcelona and Madrid and later with the older painters of Montmartre, Paris) before he painted his masterpieces. Rabindranath Tagore, though had little formal school education, was educated at home by eminent scholars in Calcutta and later in London and was an avid reader of Indian and Western literature and an astute observer of everything that he saw during his worldwide travels even up to late in his life. That was his "preparation". Interestingly, he never received any formal art training but emerged later in life as a most successful and creative painter (nearly 2000 paintings to match his 2000 songs and innumerable poetries). It was only possible for his keen observation of works of other artists (Indian, Western, and even aboriginal). His "preparation" phase was lifelong.

Is such a preparation phase always needed for creative innovation? Chance discoveries in science are, however, not too uncommon. However, it appears that the scientists (e.g., Archimedes or Sir Isaac Newton) who made such discoveries must have been prepared mentally and intellectually to grasp the significance of these accidental events or chances. It indeed is the "prepared mind"[4] that enables creators to perceive the importance of the phenomenon they observed. It is highly likely that an "incubation phase" of ideas is needed for this "preparedness". The observation and grasping of its significance constitute what is described in psychological literature as the "Aha!" experience. Historically, the author would prefer to call this the "Eureka" experience. This is what—Wallas[3] termed illumination. In science, the hypotheses arrived at need to be proved by experimentation and that is the stage of verification of Graham Wallas.[3] It must be remembered of course that in science, not many discoveries are made accidentally (hence may lack the "Aha" or "Eureka" experience) but result from a series of conscious steps (not just subconscious incubation). Thus, the categorical staging system does not work well in all aspects of the abstract concept of creativity and a general term like "creative innovation" (as proposed by Heilman et al.)[5] may be more easy to understand. The author would try to re-examine the involved issues so far noted and suggest new thoughts.

PREREQUISITES OR PREPARATION

General Intelligence

Intelligence is supposed to be domain specific just like creativity in general. Domain-specific intelligence is difficult to assess. A cricketer who innovated the reverse swing or the reverse sweep or innovates a batting stroke for an odd ball, which is not described in cricketing books, is certainly creative. But he need not have been a "bright" boy at school. However, if you define intelligence as a measure of a person's ability to acquire the knowledge and skill that will allow them to adopt to their environment,[6] a basic level of intelligence would be a prerequisite for any creative endeavor; of course, the relationship may not be a linear one. Barron and Harrington[7] found a weak relationship between creativity of architects and their IQ. They concluded that above an IQ of about 120, the IQ does not predict creativity as much as it does if the IQ is below 120. This suggests that there is an IQ threshold. A person needs to be above the threshold to be intelligent enough to learn and have sufficient knowledge about the domain of their activity. Thus, intelligence is a necessary but not sufficient component of creativity.

Knowledge and Special Talents

A person may have a specific cognitive disorder, e.g., a learning disorder like dyslexia or even autism, but can have creative talents in another field even to the level of a creative genius. Such people are often referred as "savants" and while the possible brain mechanisms of savants would not be discussed at this stage, some concrete examples from history would highlight the point. Writings of Leonardo da Vinci, examined recently,[8] suggest that he probably had developmental dyslexia. However, the world has yet to see such an expression of multidomain creativity as observed in Leonardo. Both Picasso and Einstein most likely suffered from learning disorders.

Thus, general intelligence (which may be unaltered in dyslexia) or what Spearman[9] called the "g" factor alone cannot explain specific disabilities or specific talents and several theories have placed more emphasis on special factors called the "S" factor.

Weisberg[10] concluded that domain-specific knowledge is a prerequisite for creativity. This knowledge in human is generally stored in the posterior neocortex in the region of the inferior parietal lobule (Broadman areas 39 and 40) and the posterior portion of the temporal lobe (area 37). Lesional studies confirm that these areas are important in mediating many higher cognitive activities such as literary skill, mathematics, and spatial computation.

BRAIN STRUCTURE–CREATIVITY RELATIONSHIP

Is it true that larger a particular brain area devoted to a function better if that function performed? Norman Geschwind[11] and his coworkers demonstrated that the left temporal planum, which mediates language, is larger than that on the right and other anatomic asymmetries exist between the right and left brains. Early in the 20th century, it was noted that several mathematicians and physicists had large parietal lobes but little research was done to document this observation until the works on Einstein's brain. Einstein himself thought that the best way to learn brain mechanisms in creativity would be to examine the brains of creative people. So, in accordance with his will, his brain was removed soon after his death in 1955 and was photographed and preserved. The brain subsequently was cut into several (as many as 240) pieces and sent to various institutions in USA and Canada. However, most pieces were lost, and reports from only two centers are available.

Fortunately, the brain was photographed before sectioning, and only in 1999 (that is 44 years after Einstein's death), the findings were made available by Witelson et al.,[12] working at McMaster University in Hamilton, Canada. The photographs show a striking feature. The posterior ramus of the sylvian fissure instead of turning upward behind the postcentral sulcus to divide the inferior parietal lobule into supramarginal and angular gyri actually got continued with the caudal end of the postcentral sulcus. Consequently, Einstein had a large undivided inferior parietal lobule—the area which specializes for mathematical skills and spatial computation. However, this work was criticized by Foundas and her coworkers[13] and thus Einstein's exceptional creativity cannot solely be accounted for by the undivided large inferior parietal lobule. Histological studies on the brain, however, were available earlier (1985).

Diamond et al.[14] performed a histological analysis of both right and left Broadman's area 9 (superior frontal gyrus) and area 39 (angular gyrus) of Einstein's brain and found that compared to controls, area 39 of Einstein's brain contained a higher glial cell-neuron ratio. They thought that this unusual ratio was a response by the glial cells to greater neuronal metabolic need which could have been related to Einstein's unusual conceptual power. This report was severely criticized for methodological reasons. Kantha[15] posited that Einstein had developmental dyslexia and hypothesized that the abnormality reported by Diamond et al.[14] may have been related to Einstein's dyslexia rather than his genius. Heilman and his coworker[5] much later suggested that the high index of glial cells found in Einstein's brain might have indicated a high degree of connectivity. This, as we shall examine later in the article, is closely related to creativity.

PHENOMENON OF PARADOXICAL FUNCTIONAL FACILITATION

Geschwind and Galaburda[16] suggested that the delay in development of left hemisphere (as occurs in dyslexia) may allow the right hemisphere, that mediates spatial computation, to become highly specialized. Einstein's creativity was heavily dependent on spatial reasoning and abnormal development of left hemisphere may have allowed the right hemisphere to become highly specialized for spatial computation. De novo development of artistic or musical skills (which resides in the right hemisphere) has also been described in several patients with left hemispheric dysfunction including frontotemporal dementia.[17] This somewhat paradoxical observation can be explained on the basis of the theory of paradoxical functional felicitation proposed by Kapur.[18] This, Kapur[18] thought, occurs as a compensatory augmentation occurring as a specific manifestation of central nervous system (CNS) plasticity. The present author wishes to call this "Reverse Diaschisis". In diaschisis, as first described by von Monakow in 1914, reduced function of one brain area leads to reduced function of a remote brain area to which it is anatomically connected. The reverse occurs here. Dysfunction of the left brain leads to disinhibited functioning of the right brain.

FURTHER OBSERVATIONS ON BRAIN STRUCTURE AND CREATIVITY RELATION

We do not know whether all creative people harbor specific anatomic differences in areas needed for specialized knowledge. However, specialized knowledge might also depend on a region's cellular organization and neurochemicals found in this region. It may be hypothesized that more neurons that a person is endowed with, greater their ability to learn and store knowledge. However, on the other hand, experimental animals, who were put in an enriched environment and who could learn better, had a thicker cerebral cortex with an increase in number of the dendritic spines[19] that are critical for neuronal connectivity and storage of knowledge. Connectivity thus seemed the most important prerequisite for the creative brain to develop. As we age, our creativity generally diminishes—not so much because of reduction in number of nerve cells but due to reduction in number of synapses, thereby reducing connectivity. The prerequisites discussed in this section prepare the brain for creative concepts and output which in turn is dependent on several factors accounting for creative innovation (incubation and illumination stages of creativity of Graham Wallas).[8]

CREATIVE INNOVATION

Several factors may contribute:

- *Divergent thinking*: Thinking "out of the box" is a major part of creative conceptualization. Novel understanding of a problem and seeking and expressing an orderly relationship is the hallmark of creative conceptualization. Simply speaking, a creative person needs to take a different direction from the prevailing modes of thought or expression, which is called divergent thinking.

  Oliver Zangwell[20] suggested that frontal lobe dysfunction would disrupt divergent thinking. There might be two components to divergent thinking—disengagement and developing alternative solutions. In order to find a creative solution to a problem that has remained unsolved, a person must alter the way by which people have previously attempted to solve the problem. The frontal lobes are essential for this disengagement and shift to new avenues for solution. Cognitive perseveration, the inability to set or change the form of an activity, is often observed following frontal lobe injuries or frontal lobectomies.[20] How the frontal lobes accomplish this, however, remains unknown. Pandya and Kupers[21] demonstrated that the frontal lobes have strong connection to the polymodal and supramodal regions of the temporal and parietal lobes. Perhaps, these connections are important for inhibiting the activated networks that store semantically similar information while exciting or activating the semantic conceptual networks that have been only weakly activated or not activated at all. Activation of these remote networks might be important in developing the alternative solution, so important in divergent thinking.

- *Is subtle frontal lobe dysfunction a necessity for creative innovation?—a hypothesis*: As discussed earlier, frontal dysfunction is detrimental to the creative process. However, the present author feels that some degree of perseverative behavior is needed for creative output as creative scientists and artists are found to produce voluminous output of thematically similar works. However, the dysfunction must be of a subtle nature.

  Claude Monet made some thirty odd paintings of one cathedral in Rome in different weather and lighting conditions.

  Furthermore, especially for creative artists and men of letters, some disinhibition of thought process is often needed. Often, emotions and feeling lose all boundaries in writings and use of colors, which become more and more vibrant and brush strokes more and more bold. When Tagore wrote "I shall flood you with the waves of love" or even "death is like divine to me"—surely these are examples of disinhibited emotion of love and surrendering to God (the present author's translations).

  Thinking a little broadly, it seems likely that subtle frontal dysfunction would be conducive toward divergent thinking and toward novelty seeking behavior and suppression of latent inhibition, as we shall discuss later.

  The other side of the coin is of course, the disinhibited character and manners seen in many poets and artists. Alcoholism, drug use, unkempt appearance, and sexual promiscuity, resulting from disinhibited behavior, are unhelpful to the society. It seems to the present author that the relationship between frontal disinhibitory behavior and creativity is in the form of an inverted "U".
- *Latent inhibition*: It may be described as the capacity of the brain to filter from conscious awareness stimuli previously perceived as irrelevant[22] as measured by various behavioral tests in humans and animals. This construct figures prominently in numerous theories of schizophrenia and it has been demonstrated that reduced latent inhibition is associated in psychotic states or psychotic susceptibility as well as high dopamine (DA) levels.[23] Much of the phenomenology of psychoses includes the formation of association between unrelated or irrelevant stimuli and this has led some researchers[24,25] to speculate that creativity, which involves "original recombinant ideation", may

involve a reduction in latent inhibition. In essence, looking a little broadly, reduced latent inhibition might enhance divergent thinking.

- *Novelty seeking*: Creative people are in general novelty seekers. However, creativity should not be equated always with novelty. If one wears a red shoe in one foot and a green shoe in the other, that is novel but not creative. As the result would be an eyesore and not an esthetic one. Still, novelty in concept is a result of divergent or "out of box" thinking. As mentioned earlier, creative artists, writers, and composers/musicians show a high incidence of alcoholism.[26] On one hand, this suggests a frontally disinhibited behavior and socially looked down upon. However, there is a finer neuro-psycho-pharmacologic side as well. There is some evidence that exposure to novelty activates the mesolimbic DA system of the brain.[27] Increased DA activity is highly rewarding and contributes to the illumination (Aha !) stage of creativity. The densities of DA receptors and transporters in the amygdala (the seat of emotions in humans) are low in alcohol abusers.[28] Hence, alcoholics use alcohol to stimulate DA release from such reduced number of receptors to get the "kick". In the same way, novel ideas stimulate the same receptors to generate the "Aha"! or "Eureka" sensation or feeling.

  Support for the DA hypothesis might come from the case described by Schrag and Trimble[29] where a man with Parkinson's disease (a DA-deficient state) developed previously nonexistent poetic talents (leading to publication and prizes) soon after starting a DA agonist treatment. In other words, he became creative. Moreover, as this patient had left dominant parkinsonism, it seems he had a right dominant pathology. Hence, stimulation of the right brain produced poetic creativity by disinhibiting the left brain which houses the language function. This is similar to the cases described by Miller and others[30] where left brain pathologies like frontotemporal dementias disinhibited right brain function like artistic talents.
- *Connectivity and creativity: Hemispheric dichotomy or harmony*—Creative conceptualization and creative output (incubation and illumination) have already been mentioned in relation to the observations made in Einstein's brain. The brain is organized in a modular fashion—several modules (neural networks) house different talents and capacities. Thus, the understanding, development, and expression of orderly relationship (that is what creativity is all about) might require communication between these modules.

  The strongest evidence for brain modularity is hemispheric localization of functions. The left brain stores language function, motor control of skilled movements, categorical processing, and arithmetic skills. The right brain houses spatial cognition, spatial imagery, face and object recognition, coordinates coding and emotional communication.[31] If you look at any creative work, you may find a harmonious and coordinated functioning of both the hemispheres. Take the simple example of a car driver in a narrow, congested busy road. He needs to be a skillful driver (a left brain function) to have his car unscratched and at the same time have a good spatial concept of the street plan (a right brain function), to choose the path of least resistance to reach his destination in time.

Leonardo da Vinci, excelled in drawing and painting, needed the executive skill of drawing/painting (a left brain function) as well as spatial imagery (a right brain function). He made anatomical and architectural drawing (conceptualization needing right brain and skill needing left brain functions) and made arithmetic calculations (left brain) to support his engineering skills. Einstein was a brilliant mathematician (left brain) but built his theories (relativity and gravitational) on spatially imagined concepts (right brain). Tagore excelled in language (left brain) and in painting (skill from left brain and visual imagery from right brain). So, harmonious functioning of both hemispheres in unison is essential for creative output. Connectivity, thus, is of paramount importance, and the principal structure subserving this connectivity between the two hemispheres is the corpus callosum. Callosal disconnection destroys creativity.[32] However, in addition to having this interhemispheric connectivity, intrahemispheric connectivity is of no less importance. Rabindranath Tagore exhibited multidomain creative excellence. Not only did he excel in poetry and song writing, he showed exceptional talents in prose writing, music, and visual art. In retrospect, he certainly had highly developed domain-specific neural networks in his right brain (in addition to left brain language skills) which obviously were highly interconnected (intrahemispheric connectivity). Such types of individual would be very rare to find and hence no domain-specific lesional studies (within one hemisphere) are available. It is a pity that we have no knowledge about the networking morphology of Tagore's brain. Spearman[9] suggested that creative ideas result from the combination of two or more ideas that have been previously isolated. Or in other words, developing inter- and intrahemispheric connectivity. Novelty and divergent thinking result from utilizing a new neural circuitry than what had been previously used and it may well lie in the other hemisphere.

When Einstein could not solve the mass-energy relationship through detailed mathematical calculations (utilizing his left brain), he took recourse to spatial thinking and computation (right brain function) to solve the mystery and then went back to mathematics. Einstein's creativity was related to his enhanced intra- and interhemispheric connectivity.

SYNESTHESIA AND CREATIVITY: AN EXTENSION OF THE CONNECTIVITY CONCEPT

It is said that Richard Feynman, the Novel prize winning physicist and famous for his very novel and innovative concepts, often started with abstract visual representation of his ideas, which he subsequently translated into mathematical terms. Apparently, the architecture of the networks supporting his visual representation permitted him the manipulative freedom to escape conventional formulations, thereby providing the basis for creative innovation. To the present author, this phenomenon in Richard Feynman sounds very much like synesthetic thought processing. Synesthesia, a positive neurological phenomenon that occurs from early childhood, affects 4% of the population.[33] An otherwise healthy individual has automatic and involuntary experiences in one sensory modality when a different sensory modality is stimulated. It is different for each synesthetic, and examples of these long-term discrete pairings can be simple such as the day "Tuesday" or the letter "F" triggering the experience of light pink, or more complex such as the sound of a middle "C" played on a piano triggering the sensation of a long green solid block spanning in space or the taste of salty burnt chicken. Synesthesia had frequently been reported among poets, novelists, artists, and musicians such as Rimband, Baudelaire, Kandinsky, Nabokov, Scriabin, Messiaen, and Heckney.[33] Theories of its neurological basis include hyperconnectivity[34] or diminished feedback between unimodal sensory areas of the cortex and polymodal integration areas in the temporal lobe.[35] Interestingly, synesthetics perform better on tests of creativity similar to divergent thinking and those who pursue artistic lifestyle often report needing to communicate with these unusual visual experience, through another medium. Olivier Messiaen wrote "...whenever I hear music or even if I read music, I see colors."[36] The present author has a feeling that Rabindranath Tagore probably was a synesthetic as well. He did make a vague comment about it in his conversation with Rani Chanda (*Alapcharita Rabindranath*). Tagore took to painting quite late in life. All his life, he wrote poetry and songs. The present author argues that when he started painting, his own songs and poems continually "played" in his brain (and new songs/poetry as well, as he composed several new ones even while he was deeply engaged in painting) to give rise to color sensation. His paintings are hence so vibrant in color with bold brush strokes and bold borders. He has, of course, red–green color blindness (protanopic probably) and the color "true" red is conspicuously absent in his paintings.

But what may be the possible mechanism of association of synesthesia with creativity. Synesthetes have additional neural activation during the synesthetic experience over and above activation involved in typical mental imagery. For example, the angular gyrus shows greater activation in synesthetes[37] and consistent with its strategic location at the crossroads between the temporal, parietal, and occipital lobes, and is likely to serve in the function of cross-modal association. The synesthetic coactivation in different sensory modes creates a de-focus of attention from just the trigger sensation to another sensation. Broadened cortical activation is also correlated with an increase in ideation productivity and importantly a decrease in fixation that stunts creative thought in typical population.[38] This could explain how synesthetes, who experience an excess coactivation in different areas of cortex continually in everyday life, can have a propensity for high creative thinking abilities. This is significant to the understanding of synesthesia, and creative cognition, because the ability to use one network architecture to represent another is hypothesized to enable escape of constraints in the original network and lead to novel association, solutions, and subsequent pattern formation. The present author feels this is what Heilman et al.[5] referred to as "creativity by metaphor".

AROUSAL, MOOD, AND CREATIVITY

Several scientists have mentioned that they had had the experience of solving many complex scientific problems during sleep or when they were either falling asleep or on awakening. Ramanujam, the great mathematician, is known to having solved mathematical problems during sleep. Kekule, who described the hexagonal structure of the benzene ring, is said to have dreamt of a snake chasing its own tail and Crick is said to have dreamt of two interlocking snakes before he conceptualized the double helix structure of the DNA. How far these are true is not really known and neither it is known how Freud would have interpreted such dreams! The Spanish anatomist Ramon Y Cajal[39] in his book, "Advice for a Young Investigator" advised resting, if a difficult solution cannot be arrived at. High cortical arousal induced by stress is often associated with conscious attempts at problem solving. But this high arousal might suppress the emergence of remote associations which forms the neural basis of divergent thinking and creativity. Lower degree of cortical arousal might allow unusual association to become manifest facilitating creative thinking.[40]

Kraeplin in 1921 was perhaps the first to note that manic-depressive psychosis was often associated with enhanced creativity.[10] Several investigations have reported that many of our most creative writers, composers, painters, and scientists have suffered with depression either bipolar or monopolar. Among the eminent artists showing most probably manic-depression or cyclothymic symptoms were—E Dickinson, Ernest Hemingway, N Gogol, A Strindberg, V Woolf, Lord Byron, JW Goethe, Vincent van Gogh, F Goya, G Donizetti, GF Handel, O Klemperer, G Mahler, R Schuman, and H Wolf.[41]

During his blue period (starting in 1901), Picasso was also very depressed (blue is the color of depression). There are indications that he was looking for a more personal and intimate style, his finances were meagre, and he was worried about his future lest he has to face the miseries like Van Gogh or Cezzane.[42] Rabindranath Tagore suffered from depression from an early age. This is apparent in some of his writings, in his biographies (e.g., that by Prabhat Kumar Mukherjee) and his conversations with Rani Chanda (*Alapcharita Rabindranath*). He lost his mother early, lost his very close sister-in-law, then his own wife, one son and one daughter, his very favorite nephew Balendranath, and lastly in old age his dear grandson. He faced criticisms from his contemporaries, had severe financial difficulty for the educational institution he established, was much aggrieved by the sufferings of his countrymen under the British rule, and was worried for his differences of opinion with other national leaders like Gandhi. Yet he embraced his misfortunes, never blamed anybody and wrote "O cruel Almighty; whatever you have done is good for me; an incense stick does not emit any fragrance unless burnt; a candle does not give light unless lighted" (present author's translation). His life is a vivid example of creating in the midst of depression. How can arousal, relaxation, and depression be related to creativity? The possible link appears to be changes in level of neurotransmitters, and norepinephrine (NE) in particular which is reduced both during sleep, relaxation, and depression. How this may be related to the creative process is discussed in the next section.

CATECHOLAMINES AND CREATIVITY

The roles of two catecholamines have been discussed in relation to creativity—DA and NE. Both are related in the sense that NE is a product of DA metabolism. The possible role of DA had already been discussed in relation to novelty seeking.

As discussed in the previous section, to creativity as stress is associated with high brain NE level. On the other hand, sleep and relaxation being associated with a low NE state enhance creativity. Faigel[43] showed that students taking propranolol, a centrally acting β-blocker reducing effect of NE on neurons, improved performance of students taking the Scholastic Aptitude Test (SAT), which tests both crystallized knowledge and fluid reasoning, that NE modulates cognitive flexibility had also been shown in experiments. That NE modulates involving problem solving after pretreatment with ephedrine and propranolol,[44] and also comparing effect of propranolol and nadolol, a peripherally acting β-blocker.[45] Only central β-adrenergic blockade increased cognitive flexibility.

The locus coeruleus (LC) is the richest source which provides NE output to the cortex. Aston-Jones et al.[46] posited that high levels of tonic LC activity, which increases the levels of NE in the cortex, are important for "monitoring and attending to external stimuli and increasing behavioral responsiveness to unexpected and novel stimuli". It is thus needed for the "flight or fight" activities. It follows, therefore, that low levels of LC activity would enhance creative cognition and outputs.

The frontal lobes appear to be able to exert an inhibitory influence on the LC.[47] Hence, frontal disinhibitory behaviors would be nonconducive for creative activity. On the other hand, the author had already postulated that a subtle degree of frontal dysfunction is conducive for creative activity. How does one solve this puzzle? The present author feels that the relationship between frontal disinhibition and LC activity is inverted U-shaped. At low levels of disinhibition, LC activity diminishes providing reduced levels of NE to cortex which facilitates orderly distributed representations (thus enhancing creative thinking) and high level of frontal disinhibition would enhance LC activity with high NE level at cortex which is nonconducive for creativity. An analogy can be drawn from the relationship between mood and creativity concept of where the relationship is also in an inverted "U" form. Elevation of mood facilitates creativity to a certain point beyond which extreme increase has an adverse effect on achievements.[48] Perhaps, the same is true for depression as well.

CREATIVE COGNITION AND OUTPUT: AN ALL EMBRACING CONCEPTUAL HYPOTHESIS

The concept of creativity is an abstract one—a phenomenon of the mind, but it has to be a function of the brain. However, because of its abstract nature and for the fact that creativity is largely a domain-specific behavior, Jacksonian concept of cerebral localization of neurological function and phenomenon cannot be applied here. The seat of creativity is likely to remain undetermined. Neuropsychological tests for creativity can only give a very partial insight into man's creativity and such tests have not been applied to really creative people as we recognize them. Hence, approach to conceptualization has to be somewhat anecdotal as has been made in this chapter. However, based on known functions of different brain areas, a working model of flow of thought processing which ultimately leads to creative cognition and output can perhaps be hypothesized. The output in most forms of creative works is one of problem solving and thinking broadly artists and men of literature possibly make the same endeavor as well.

So we can assume facing a problem to be the trigger for creative cognition to begin. It may be suggested that this process starts in the prefrontal lobe. But surely, along with this, a curious phenomenon also occurs in the prefrontal cortex whereby there is simultaneous subtle suppression of frontal inhibitory behavior. The neural circuitry involved would be complex and it would be difficult to hypothesize on this at the present stage. The creative cognitive thoughts can thus flow uninterrupted because of disinhibition of frontal control on divergent (out of box) thinking and aided by suppression of latent inhibition, as highlighted earlier in this chapter. The latter makes room for the divergently thinking mind to choose from several different paths to problem solving (including unconventional ones) which were not available earlier to others due to frontal inhibitory behavior. This conceptual phenomenon leads to development of novelty—a core feature of most creative works. Continuing challenge from divergent thinking during the creative process would enhance intra- and interhemispheric connectivity (possibly through generation of neurotropic factors with establishment of new synapses) which would further augment divergent thinking and thus self-rewarding. The frontally generated creative cognitive flow would certainly be enriched by other brain areas (like from memory, emotion, output from areas for artistic and mathematical talent, etc.) and then would finally lead to creative output. This likely is also an essentially frontally governed phenomenon. **Flowchart 1** summarizes the present author's hypothetical view on the generation of creative output from thought initiation to the final result.

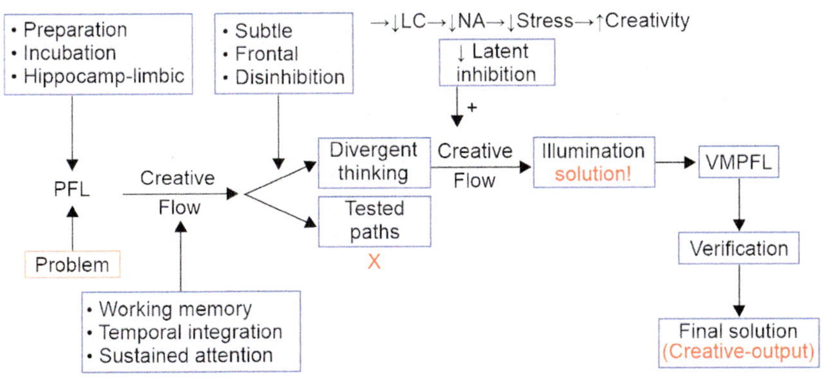

FLOWCHART 1: Creative flow: A hypothesis.

(PFL: prefrontal lobe; LC: locus coeruleus; NA: noradrenaline; VMPFL: ventromedial prefrontal lobe)

Source: Reprinted with modifications from Chakravarty A. The creative brain—revisiting concepts. Med Hypotheses. 2010;74(3):606-12.

CONCLUDING REMARKS

Why would a clinical neurologist be interested in the process of creativity which essentially is a mental phenomenon having no proved discrete cerebral localization not following the Jacksonian concept that all neurological phenomenon can be localized to a specific area of the brain? Thinking neurologically is a creative act in the same way that thinking artistically, musically, or scientifically is creative. The profession of clinical neurology is an intrinsically artistic endeavor. Finding unity among myriads of diverse symptoms is certainly a creative task as highlighted early in this article. Neurologists may not be able to say where the artistic process is located in the brain, but they can at least have the pleasure of feeling what it is to be creative.

Much of what we have learnt about creativity in general is based on hypotheses. It would be a daunting task even for a creative brain to unravel the mystery of creativity. The present author would tend to disagree with Albert Einstein's view that studying the brains of creative people at postmortem would be helpful. Lots lie in functioning rather than structure. A theoretical solution might be to perform functional imaging studies of creative people at work. This seems impractical at the present state of our knowledge and available technology. One cannot ask an artist to paint or a mathematician to solve a puzzle while lying inside the gantry of an MR scanner. There is certainly a limit to human understanding of the "Language of God".

REFERENCES

1. Meyers H, Gerstman R. Creativity. New York: Palgrave Macmillan; 2008.
2. Bronowski J. Science and human values. New York: Harper and Row; 1972.
3. Wallas G. The art of thought. New York: Harcourt Brace; 1926.
4. Kuhn TS. The structure of scientific revolutions, 3rd edition. Chicago: University of Chicago Press; 1996.
5. Heilman KM, Nadeau SE, Beversdorf DQ. Creative innovation: Possible brain mechanism. Neurocase. 2003;9:369-79.
6. Sternberg RJ. The concept of intelligence and its role in lifelong learning and success. Am Psychol. 1997;52:1030-7.
7. Barron F, Harrington DM. Creativity, intelligence and personality. Ann Rev Psychol. 1981;32:439-76.
8. Rosstad A. Leonardo da Vinci – a dyslectic genius? Tidsskr Nor Laegeforen. 2002;122:2887-94.
9. Spearman C. General intelligence. Objectively determined and measured. Am J Psychol. 1905;15:210-93.
10. Weisberg RW. Creativity and knowledge. A challenge to theories. In: Sternberg RJ (Ed). Handbook of Creativity. Cambridge: Cambridge University Press; 1999. pp. 226-50.
11. Geschwind N, Levitsky W. Human brain: Left right asymmetries in temporal speech region. Science. 1968;161:186-7.
12. Witelson SF, Kigor DL, Harvey T. The exceptional brain of Albert Einstein. Lancet. 1999;353:2149-53.
13. Foundas AL, Faulhaber JR, Kulynach JJ, Browning CA, Weinberger DR. Hemispheric and gender differences in sylvian fissure morphology: A quantitative approach using volumetric MRI. Neuropsychiatry Neuropsychol Behav Neurol. 1999;12:1-10.
14. Diamond MC, Scheibel AB, Murphy GM Jr, Harvey T. On the brain of a scientist: Albert Einstein. Exp Neurol. 1985;88:198-204.

15. Kantha SS. Albert Einstein's dyslexia and the significance of Broadman Area 39 of his left cerebral cortex. Med Hypothes. 1992;37:119-22.
16. Geschwind N, Garabuda AM. Cerebral lateralization. Biological mechanisms, sociations and pathology. A hypothesis and programme for research. Arch Neurol. 1985;42:425-59, 634-59.
17. Pollak TA, Mulvenna CM, Lythgoe M. De novo artistic behavior following brain injury. In: Bogousslavsky J, Hennerici MG (Ed). Neurological Disorders in Famous Artists – Part 2. Basel: Karger; 2007. pp. 75-88.
18. Kapur N. Paradoxical functional facilitation in brain – behavior research. A critical review. Brain. 1997;119:1775-90.
19. Rosenzweig MR, Bennett EL. Psychobiology of plasticity: Effects of training and experience on brain and behavior. Behav Brain Res. 1996;78:57-66.
20. Zangwell OL. Psychological deficits associated with frontal lobe lesions. Int J Neurol. 1996;5:395-402.
21. Pandya DN, Kuypers HG. Cortico-cortical connections in the Rhesus monkey. Brain Res. 1969;13:13-36.
22. Lubow RE, Moore AU. Latent inhibition: the effect of non-reinforced pre-exposure to the conditional stimulus. J Comp Physiol Psychol. 1959:52:415-9.
23. Gray JA. Integrating schizophrenia. Schizophr Bull. 1998;24:249-66.
24. Carson SH, Peterson JB, Higgins DM. Decreased latent inhibition is associated with increased creative achievement in high functioning individuals. J Pers Soc Psychol. 2003;85:499-506.
25. Flaherty AW. Frontotemporal and dopaminergic control idea generation and creative drive. J Comp Neurol. 2005;493:147-53.
26. Post F. Creativity and Psychopathology. A study of 291 world famous men. Br J Psychiat. 1994;165:22-34.
27. Bardo MT, Donohew RL, Harrington NG. Psychobiology of novelty seeking and drug seeking behaviour. Behav Br Res. 1996;77:23-43.
28. Tupala E, Hall H, Bergstorm K, Sarkioja T, Räsänen P, Mantere T, et al. Dopamine D(2)/D(3) – receptor and transporter densities in nucleus acumbens and amygdala of type 1 and 2 alcoholics. Mol Psychiatry. 2001;6:261-7.
29. Schrag A, Trimble M. Poetic talent unmasked by treatment of Parkinson's Disease. Mov Disord. 2001;16:1175-76.
30. Miller BL, Yener G, Akdal G. Artistic patterns in dementia. J Neurol Sci (Turk). 2005;3:245-49.
31. Heilman KM, Blonder LX, Bowars D, Crucian GP. Neurological disorders and emotional dysfunction. In: Borod JC (Ed). The Neuropsychology of Emotions. Series in affective science. New York: Oxford University Press; 2000. pp. 367-412.
32. Lewis RT. Organic signs, creativity, and personality characteristics of patients following cerebral commissurotomy. Clin Neuropsychol. 1979;1:29-33.
33. Mulvenna CM. Synesthesia, the Arts and Creativity: A neurological connection. In: Bogousslavasky J, Hennirici MG (Ed). Neurological Disorders in Famous Artists – Part 2. Basel: Karger; 2007. pp. 206-22.
34. Ramachandran VS, Hubbard EM. Synaesthesia – a window into perception, thought and language. J Conscious Stud. 2001;8:3-34.
35. Esterman M, Verstynen T, Ivry RB, Robertson LC. Coming unbound: disrupting automatic integration of synaesthetic colour and graphemes by TMS of right parietal lobe. J Cogn Neurosci. 2006;l8:1570-76.
36. Cytowic R. The man who tested shapes. New York: Putnam; 1993.
37. Weiss PH, Zilles K, Fink GR. When Visual perception causes feeling: Enhanced cross-modal processing in grapheme-color synesthesia. Neuroimage. 2005;28:859-68.
38. Howard-Jones PA, Murray S. Ideational productivity, focus of attention and context. Creativity Res J. 2003;15:153-66.
39. Ramon Y Cajal S. Advice for a Young Investigator (Translated by Swanson N and Swanson LW). Cambridge: MIT Press; 1999.

40. Eysenck HJ. Genius: The natural history of creativity. Cambridge: Cambridge University Press. 1995.
41. Janka Z. Artistic creativity and bipolar mood disorder. Orv Hetil. 2004;145:1709-18.
42. Hilton T. Picasso. London: Thames and Hudson; 2003.
43. Faigel HC. The effects of beta blockades on stress induced cognitive dysfunction in adolescents. Clin Pediatr. 1991;30:446-48.
44. Beversdorf DQ, Hughes JD, Steinberg BA, Lewis LB, Heilman KM. Noradrenergic modulation of cognitive flexibility in problem solving. Neuroreport. 1999;10:2763-67.
45. Broome DMW, Cheever DC, Hughes JB, Beversdorf DQ. Effects of central and peripheral beta-blockers on non-adrenergic modulation of cognitive flexibility. J Cogn Neurosci. 2000;12:S105.
46. Aston-Jones G, Chiang C, Alexinsky T. Discharge of locus coeruleus neurons in behaving rats and monkeys suggests a role in vigilance. Prog in Br Res. 1991;88:501-20.
47. Sara SJ, Herve-Minvielle A. Inhibitory influence of frontal cortex on locus coeruleus neurons. Proc Nat Acad Sci. 1995;92:6032-6.
48. Janka Z. The impact of mood alterations on creativity. Ideggyogy Sz. 2006;59:236-40.

(Reprinted with modifications from Chakravarty A. The creative brain--revisiting concepts. Med Hypotheses. 2010 Mar;74(3):606-12.)

CHAPTER

3

Fundamentals of Art Neuroscience

INTRODUCTION

Visual art, as with all other arts, is spontaneously created only by homo sapiens and is present in various forms and extents in almost all societies today. Diving deep into the roots of art from cognitive, neurological, genetic, evolutionary, archaeological, and biological perspectives is essential for the full understanding of why we have art, and what art is about. The cognitive basis of art is symbolic, abstract, and differential thinking. Archaeological markers of symbolic activity by early humans are not associated with art production. There is an enormously large time gap between the activity and the appearance of sporadic art by early homo sapiens, and another large time delay before appearance of pain staking practice of art. The aesthetic aspect of art was probably not considered to be the initial impetus for creating it. On the other hand, archaeological markers suggest that the early beginnings of art are associated with development of stratified societies where external visual identifiers by way of body ornaments and decorations were used. According to Ramachandran[1]—*"the major contributing forces for the consistency in art-making are presumed to be the formation of socioculture, intragroup cooperation, increased group size, survival of skillful artisans, and favorable demographic conditions."* The biological roots of art are hypothesized to parallel aspects of our ancestry, specifically animal courtship displays, where signals of health and genetic quality are exhibited for inspection by potential mates. Viewers assess displayed art for talent, skill, communicativeness, and aesthetic-related qualities. Interdisciplinary discussions of art reflect the current approach to full understanding of the nature of art.

SOME FUNDAMENTALS OF VISUAL SCIENCE

Semir Zeki wrote in his book Inner Vision in 1999:[2]

Visual Brain

"All visual art is expressed through the brain and must therefore obey the laws of brain, whether in conception, execution and appreciation and no theory of aesthetics that is not substantially based on the activity of the brain is ever likely to be complete."

—Zeki, 1999

WHAT DO WE SEE WITH?

The obvious answer would be that we see with our eyes. This is not correct. True is that that light emitted from an object stimulates the photoreceptors in the retina, namely the rods and the cones. But no image is formed in the eyes; the signals received are only processed in the other nerve fibers and cells in the retina and are the transmitted to the visual areas of the cerebral cortex for deciphering their meaning like shape, size, and color. The eye, therefore, does not act like a pinhole camera where an inverted image is formed on the retina which the brain interprets as a properly oriented one; but in reality as a digital camera where the information gathered through vision is processed but transmitted to the brain's visual areas for proper interpretation as regards its size, shape, and color and meaning or identity. So in reality, we see the outside world and gather meaningful information about it, art or otherwise, only with the help of our brain. An artist creates his artwork utilizing his own brain in such a way that the creation would stimulate specific brain areas of the viewer for the created artwork to be appreciated and assess its aesthetic value. This indeed would be a neurological exercise and Zeki rightly called an artist a neurologist.

The visual areas of the brain needed for seeing and interpretation are principally located in the occipital areas of the brain and mostly on the medial or inner surfaces **(Fig. 1)**. Information to these is sent from the retinae of the eyes through the optic pathways. Areas V1/V2 lying on the lips of the calcarine fissure on the medial occipital surfaces receive the first information about seeing an object of vision and then sent to other adjacent areas for their interpretation. Area V3 lying above area V1/V2 can appreciate shape and size helping in identifying the object and area V4 lying below areas V1/V2 helps in recognizing the color of the object. A fifth area lying on superolateral surface of the posterior parietal cortex, called area V5, can recognize movements of an object of vision. People with a lesion in this area would be able to recognize a red car when it is static but fail to recognize it if the car is moving at a high speed. A coordinated functioning of all these areas is needed for proper viewing and correct interpretation of the viewed outside world.

In addition to these five primary visual cortical areas, there are over 70 cortical areas which are involved in visual functioning going as far forward as the frontal lobes and the cingulate gyrus. The exact functioning of all these areas is not fully known but these are probably needed to assess the detailing or finer assessment of an object of vision like differentiating between different shades of a particular color and thus help in assessing the aesthetic value of a painting or sculpture and differentiating between a "good" artwork and a "bad" one.

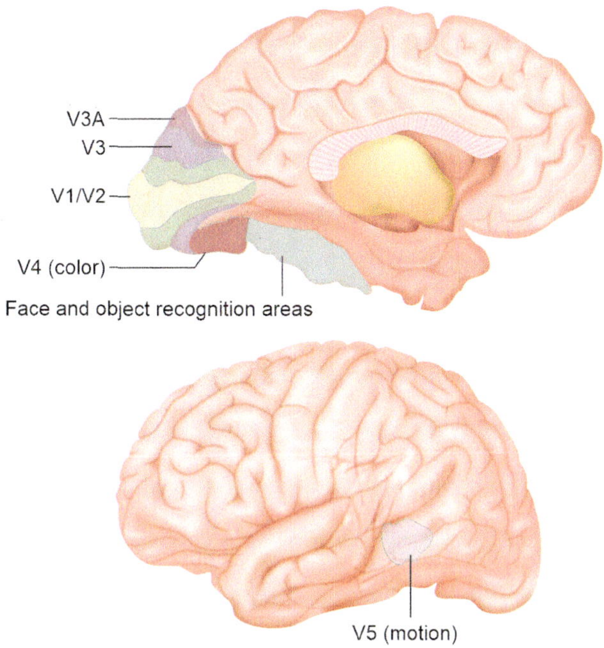

FIG. 1: Organization of the visual brain.

Zeki[2,3] conjectured that the more number of cortical areas an object of vision can stimulate the more becomes its appreciating value or aesthetic value. A movie film needs to stimulate area V5 for its proper interpretation while a still photograph need not. Thus, the appreciative value of a movie film is generally more than a still photograph. Similarly, a circular drawing would stimulate more number of neurons in area V3 than a straight line. Hence, the common saying that when you meet a woman the first three things those which strike your eyes are the eyes, the face, and lastly the breasts, because all these are rounded structures having a circular profile! In the field of art, colored paintings are generally more appreciated than black and white ones due to additional involvement of area V4. Artworks, overtly or covertly, depicting movements are more appreciative than static looking ones due to additional recruitment of area V5. This subject would be further discussed in a subsequent chapter dealing with the neurology behind Mona Lisa's smile.

Lastly, two factors need to be mentioned in relation to image viewing by the visual brain. Any object of vision can be imagined to be composed of hundreds or thousands of Dots or Pixels as referred to in modern day computer-related terminology. The brain tries to give a shape to these isolated Dots or Pixels by a special functioning, referred by Ramachandran,[1] as Grouping or Binding functioning of the brain. The simplest way for physicians is the look of the Ishihara chart used for testing color vision **(Fig. 2)**. A person with a normal color vision can easily group or bind the differently colored dots into a specific number: in the picture below it is 45.

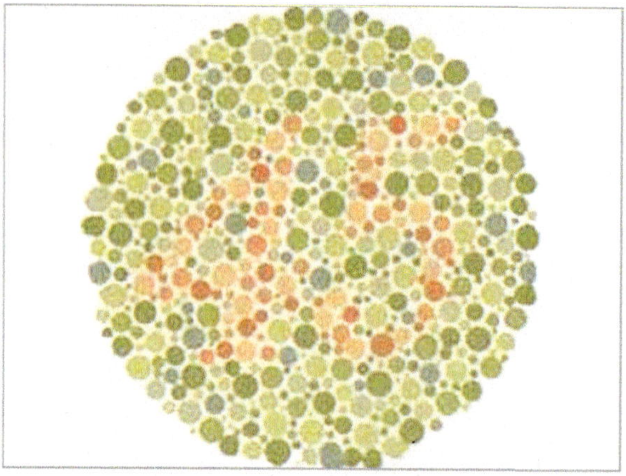

FIG. 2: Ishihara chart for color vision testing.

PRINCIPLES OF ART SCIENCE

Neuroaesthetics is a study of arts by neuroscientists. The most prominent champions of neuroaesthetics are VS Ramachandran and Seminar Zeki both of whom have made ambitious claims about their work. Ramachandran[1] says boldly that he has discovered "the key to understanding what art really is", and that his theory of art can be tested by brain imaging experiments, although he does not describe these experiments or what results the theory predicts. Zeki,[2] who originally coined the term neuroaesthetics, claims to have laid the foundations for understanding "the biological basis of aesthetic experience" and to have formulated a "neurobiological definition of art".

Ramachandran[1] writes "The purpose of art, surely, is not to depict or represent reality—for that can be accomplished very easily with a camera—but to enhance, transcend, or indeed even to distort reality... What the artist tries to do (either consciously or unconsciously) is to not really capture the essence of something but also to amplify it in order to more powerfully activate the same neural mechanisms that would be activated by the original object". But why should a distortion of reality have this effect? Ramachandran's answer, which he described as the "key to understanding what art really is", is that this is an example of a psychological effect called "peak shift" which would be expanded later in this article. He argues "there may be neurons in the brain that represent sensuous round feminine form as opposed to angular muscular form and the artist has chosen to amplify the very essence of being feminine by moving the image even further along the male/female spectrum. The result of these amplifications is a superstimulus in the domain of male/female differences."

Zeki[2] maintained that art will only become intelligible and profound once based on the workings of the brain he writes "Great art can thus be defined, in neurological terms, as that which comes closest to showing as many facets of reality, rather than the appearance, as possible...". The inestimable quality of great art is the opportunity that it is offered to give several interpretations, all of them valid. The principal difference between the views of Ramachandran and Zeki can be summarized as: does neuroscience at last hold out the promise for an intelligible and profound aesthetic theory or one that will provide the key to understanding what art really is... in Ramachandran's words "a caricature" of the reality.[1]

Ramachandran and Hirstein, in 1999,[1] described nine principles on which most artworks could be categorized which were made by the artists intentionally to increase their aesthetic values. Only three such principles would be discussed in this article:

1. *Peak shift principle*: This allows the artist to capture the details of a topic by exaggerating the details **(Figs. 3 to 6)**. The classic examples can be found in

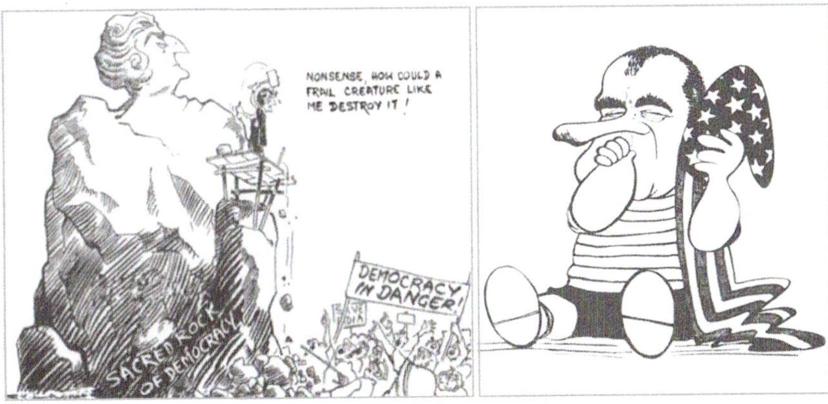
NONSENSE, HOW COULD A FRAIL CREATURE LIKE ME DESTROY IT !
DEMOCRACY IN DANGER!
SACRED ROCK OF DEMOCRACY

FIG. 3: Cartoonist art depicting peak shift.

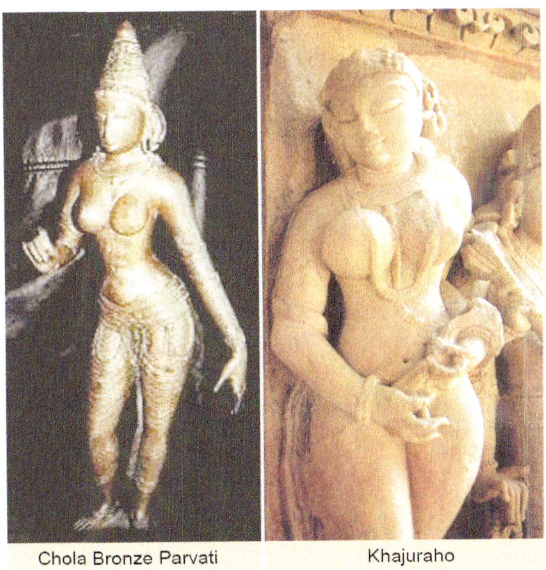
Chola Bronze Parvati
Khajuraho

FIG. 4: Ancient Indian art depicting peak shift principle.

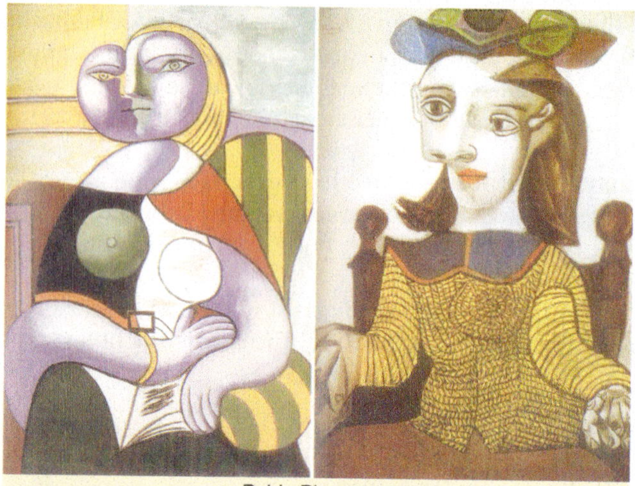

Pablo Picasso

FIG. 5: Peak shift in Cubist art.

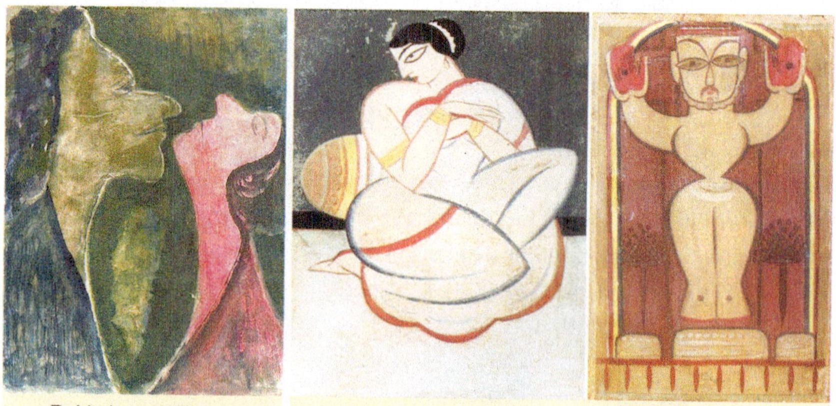

Rabindranath Tagore Jamini Roy

FIG. 6A: Peak shift in contemporary Indian art.

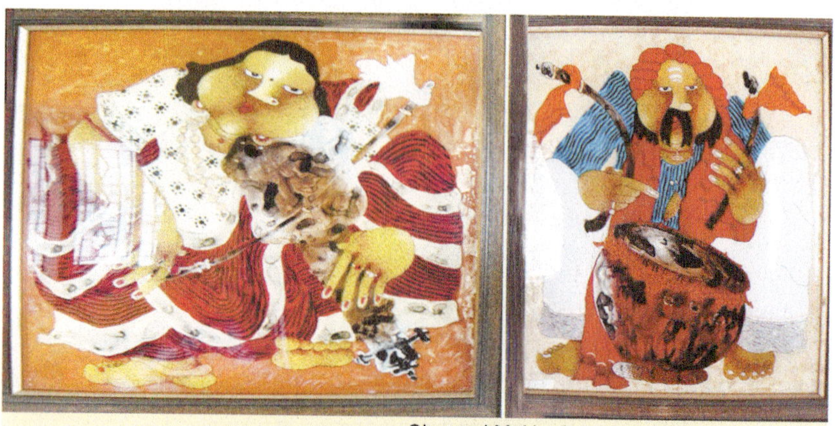

Shyamal Mukherjee

FIG. 6B: Peak shift in contemporary Indian art.

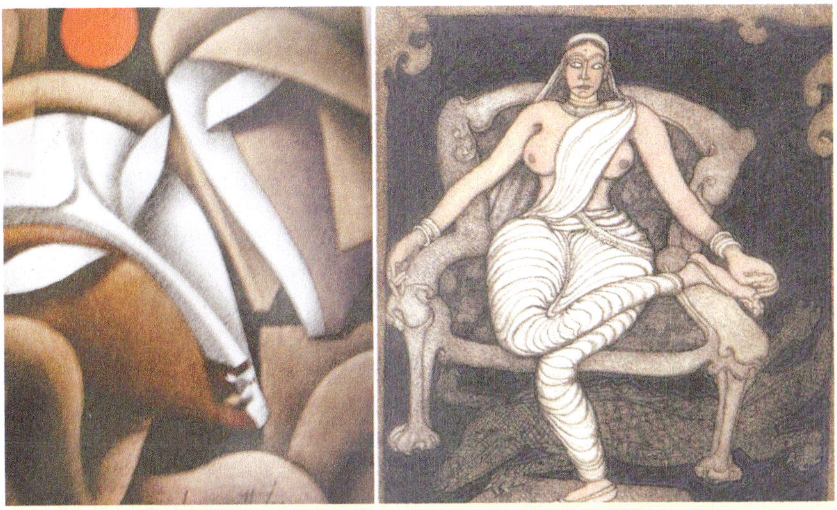

Jagannath Pal   Jogen Chowdhury

FIG. 6C: Peak shift in contemporary Indian art.

ancient artforms in the Chola Bronze sculptures as also in the stone sculptures at Khajuraho and in the Konark temple in Odisha **(Fig. 4)**. The stress had been to make feminine structures more appreciative by intentionally narrowing the waist region whereas the upper part of the bodies including the breast regions and the hip regions more prominent. This tradition had been followed by many Indian and European artists in later years and other modifications had been made keeping the fundamental technique the same. For example, Jamini Roy **(Fig. 6A)** not only made the waist regions narrower but also extended the eye lines beyond the facial outline which added a special and his signature technique to increase the painting's aesthetic values **(Fig. 6A)**. Tagore made a painting of a couple with hyperextension of their neck regions which would depict the intensity of love between the two. Several such examples exist and some are reproduced above, most of which would be self-explanatory how application of the peak shift principle enhances the aesthetic value of such paintings or sculptors.

The principle of peak shift owes its origin from an experiment performed in early 1930s with baby sea gulls. When blank white paper strips were shown to a group of baby sea gulls, none showed any interest. When some of the paper strips were marked with a red dot, many of the sea gulls started biting on the marked paper strips perhaps thinking some kinds of food were being served. When more than one red dots were placed on the paper strips, the responses were much more among the baby sea gulls. Exaggeration of the stimulus thus resulted in enhancement of the response or in other words the appreciative value of the stimulus. The same happens in case of artworks as explained earlier in this section. Cartoonists often employ the same technique to enhance the personality of famous people by exaggerating one portion of the body usually that of the face. Examples of cartoon drawings of Mrs Indira Gandhi and Richard Nixon with facial exaggeration are given in **Figure 3**.

2. *Visual isolation*: Here, the artist uses just a few lines to capture and express the essence of a visual concept.

    Anyone can make out the drawing of a Dove by Picasso signifying peace; similarly, a few lines in the subsequent two diagrams could be recognized as those belonging to Lord Ganesha and Mahatma Gandhi. The lines drawn are sufficient enough to stimulate area V3 for object recognition and the Fusiform gyrus for facial recognition **(Fig. 7)**.
3. *Grouping/binding function of the brain*: This had been briefly discussed earlier in this article with the example of the Ishihara chart for testing color vision. Every object could be thought to be composed of numerous dots or pixels. The artist puts these in such a way that the brain could group or bind these together to give a form which would make the viewer to appreciate it as a beautiful painting. The two illustrations given below **(Figs. 8 and 9)** would bring home this point. It is important to appreciate that this grouping or binding is not really a function of the art or the artist but essentially a function of the viewer's brain.

    A closer examination of these two paintings would reveal these to be composed of numerous dots and not lines or curves. Tagore attempted to do the same to paint a red bird sitting in its nest. This is also rare in the sense that Tagore had red-green color blindness.

    In summary, the three principles can be expressed as follows:

    In a later publication in 2010,[3] Ramachandran expressed similar views using different terminologies which include—grouping, peak shift, contrast, isolation, peekaboo or perceptual problem solving, abhorrence of coincidences, symmetry, and metaphor.

Art Neuroscience: A Summary

1. *Peak shift principle*: Brain's quest for the essentials
2. *Visual isolation*: Imaginative thinking → frontal cortical activation
3. *Grouping/binding*: Visual brain function

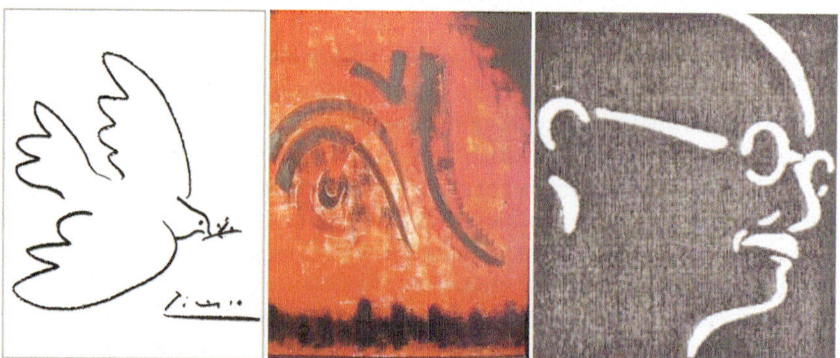

Dove Pablo Picasso | Ganesh Samir Aich | Gandhi

FIG. 7: Examples of visual isolation.

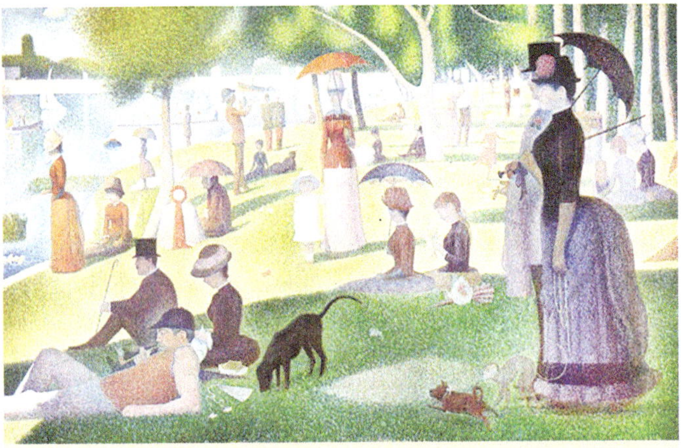

'A Sunday afternoon on the island of grand jatte' Georges Seurat

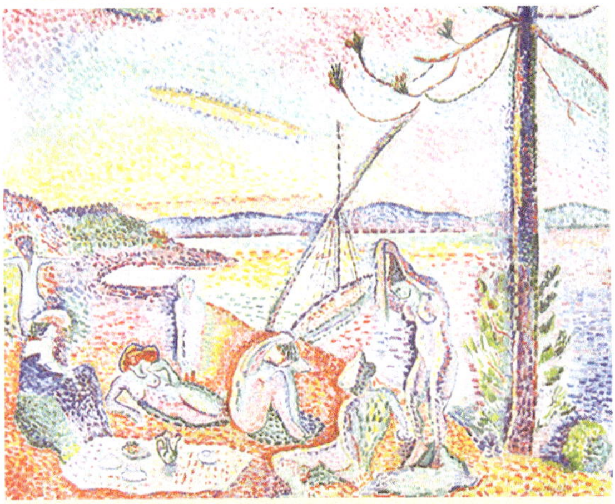

Henry Matissae

FIG. 8: Examples of grouping/binding functions of art.

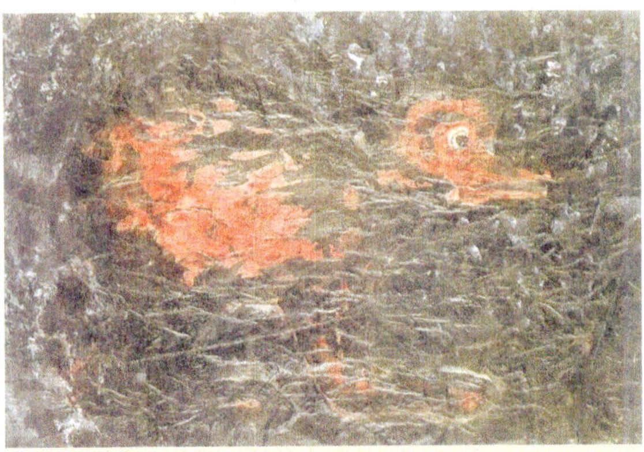

Rabindranath Tagore

FIG. 9: Grouping/binding being depicted in Tagore's painting.

SCIENCE OF PERCEPTUAL PROBLEM SOLVING AND INCOMPLETE ART FORMS

An artist can sometimes attempt to make his work more attractive by making it less visible. Look at the painting below of a nude drawn from the back without displaying the front profile at all. The viewer would automatically start imagining how the woman would look when viewed from the front. The frontal cortex would come into play for this imaginative viewing and a number of images may be thought of with different emotions in the mind of the viewer and in addition to the frontal cortex the limbic system would be activated. Interplay of these various neural pathways on viewing one single painting would automatically increase the aesthetic value of the art work. Thus, an artwork which leaves something to imagination can be much more alluring than a pinup of the same nude woman. Many people would prefer this sort of concealment because we are hardwired to love solving puzzles and perception is more like puzzle solving than most people realize **(Fig. 10)**.

Some artists often leave a work unfinished. The reason is the same. The artist wants his viewers to tax their brains to find what the artist had in mind about the unfinished body part left behind. The sculpture below would illustrate this beautifully where the viewer needs to think whether the missing limb would be in a flexed or extended position. Frontal cortical stimulation comes into play and the art work becomes more aesthetic **(Fig. 11)**.

Ramachandran did not include depiction of motion or movement in an essentially static art form. Zeki referred to this as Kinetic Art. The present author described it as Dynamism which may be overt or covert that is imaginative. This

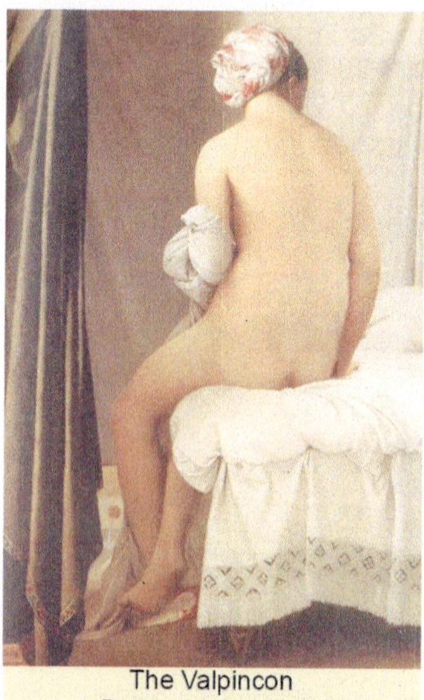

The Valpincon
Bather Ingres 1808

FIG. 10: Seen and half seen: Neuropsychology.

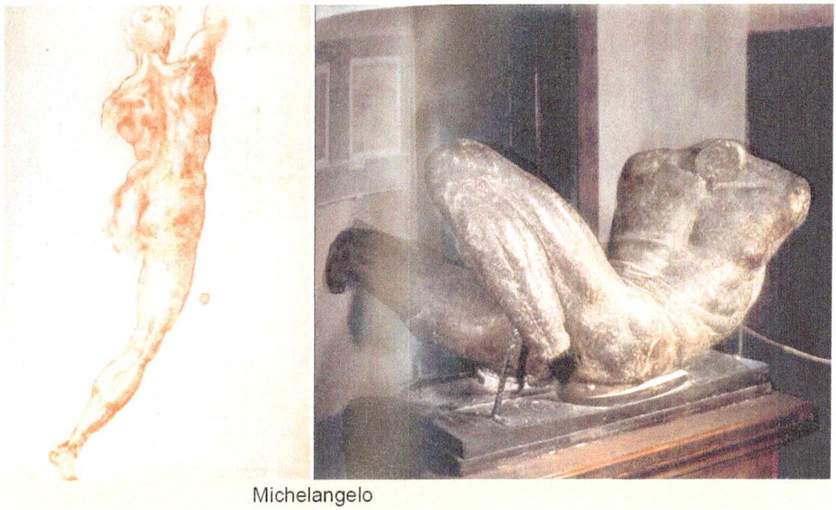

FIG. 11: Neuropsychology of unfinished art (Michelangelo's painting and sculpture).

would be discussed in a subsequent chapter in relation to Mona Lisa's smile. Such inclusion gives an added dimension to the aesthetic value of the art created.

CONCLUDING REMARKS

The author doubts very much how many artists in real life are conversant with the writings of either Zeki or Ramachandran. The principles described above are somehow ingrained in the brains of those individuals and probably culturally or genetically acquired. Innovation is the key to creativity but in practice most such innovations would tend to be one of the principles described above and indeed functions of the brain rather than that of the art. As Zeki wrote—"An artist is a neurologist" who is conscious of the fundamentals of brain functioning. Can the reverse be true as well—Is a neurologist an artist? A person, who can correlate an upgoing toe with a squint in the eye, is certainly one who finds unity in diversity and this happens to be the essence of creative thinking. If you want to see how beautiful our earth is, one needs to go out of this earth in a spaceship and then look at the earth from a distance; similarly, if you would like to see how beautiful neuroscience is, one needs to go out of neuroscience (e.g., in the world of arts) and then look at neuroscience from a distance.

REFERENCES

1. Ramachandran VS, Hirstein W. The Science of Art: A Neurological Theory of Aesthetic Experience. J Conscious Stud. 1999;6:15-51.
2. Zeki S. Inner Vision. An explanation of Art and The Brain. Oxford: Oxford University Press; 1999.
3. Ramachandran VS. Tell-Tale Brain. India: Random House; 2010.

CHAPTER

4

Mona Lisa's Smile: A Hypothesis Based on a New Principle of Art Neuroscience

INTRODUCTION

Some paintings are shrouded in mystery. The World's most famous and most viewed painting, the great master Leonardo da Vinci's (1452–1519) Mona Lisa (La Gioconda—the name in which it is displayed in Salon 16 of the Musée du Louvre, Paris), is perhaps the finest example. The long history of Mona Lisa (painted around 1502) is enigmatic—several questions have been raised and mostly remain unanswered. Why did Leonardo paint this beautiful lady? Was it really commissioned by the Italian nobleman Giocondo? Was this lady Giocondo's wife or mistress? Was Leonardo in love with her? Was she a real woman or simply drawn from the artist's imagination? Could the painting be a self-portrait of Leonardo himself drawn as a woman? Why did Leonardo left it unsigned and why he did not return it to Giocondo and kept it with him for over 10 years and took it out of Italy when he moved out to France probably in 1517? But the most intriguing mystery of all is the reason for Mona Lisa's smile—so beautifully depicted in the painting **(Fig. 1)**. Art critics have debated over years and even physicians very recently raise the question of Mona Lisa suffering from hyperlipidemia (The Times London, 6 January, 2010). Gombrich, the famous art historian commented (in his book The Story of Art)[1] that Leonardo very intelligently shaded the angles of Mona Lisa's mouth so that it gives an illusion of a smiling face. But why? In this essay, I offer a visual scientific hypothetic explanation based on a new principle of art neuroscience which I would call "Dynamism". However, before describing what I mean by dynamism in a static visual art form, I wish to write briefly on the fundamental principles of functioning of the visual brain and also on the principles of art science or the science of visual aesthetics as had been descried earlier.

PRINCIPLES OF VISUAL BRAIN FUNCTIONING

These have been adequately explained in several articles published over the last 20 years and nicely summarized in Semir Zeki's classic monograph—Inner Vision.[2]

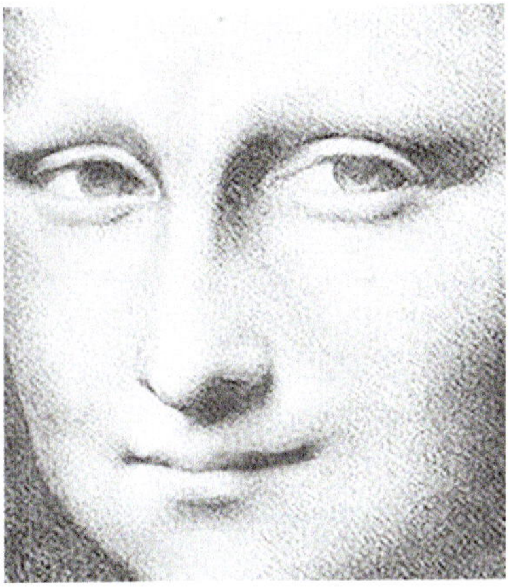

FIG. 1: BW reproduction of blown-up face of Mona Lisa (Leonardo da Vinci, 1502, Musée du Louvre, Paris).

It is important to realize that truly speaking we do not see with our eyes but with our brain. Contrary to usual belief, the eye does not act as a pinhole camera and no images are formed on the retina. Every object of vision can be assumed to consist of multiple tiny dots (or better perhaps "pixels"). Light reflected from each of these tiny dots falls on the retina and stimulates one or more retinal photoreceptors. No images are formed, but this activity from the retinal photoreceptors is transmitted to the visual brain through the retino-optic pathway where stimuli coming from individual dots of the object of vision are "grouped" or "bound" together to give rise to an image which we see. The image is formed by specific neurons of the visual brain depending on the positional directional trajectories of the individual "dots" on the object of vision—this gives the impression of shape, size, and form—a realization of two- or three-dimensional form.

Current functional neuroimaging studies indicate that there are over 70 visual areas, each with specific visual function, which are not simply localized in the occipital lobe but are spread over more anterior parts of the cortex even as far forward as the hippocampus and the prefrontal lobe. We generally talk about 5 or 6 visual areas which are relevant to clinical neurological practice.

The principal visual area V1/V2 is located on the lips of the calcarine sulcus; adjacent to it, lies area V3, needed for recognizing shape, size, and form of an object of vision; below area V3 lies area V4 which is the visual center for color vision and color is perceived by specific visual neurons in area V4 and not by retinal cones which simply transmit signals from activation by lights of specific wavelength. The most important visual area relevant to this essay is the area V5 on MT—the visual area for identifying motion in a scene of vision—which is located on the superolateral surface of brain in the posterior part of the superior temporal gyrus. The neurons in this area are direction specific in the sense that each neuron may only be stimulated by "dots" moving in any particular direction only. Light emanating (or reflected) from an object in motion (individual dots or pixels on the object) stimulates retinal photoreceptors and then this sensation of activation is first relayed to area V1/V2 and then transmitted to specific direction sensitive neurons of area V5 where motion is perceived. There is also another pathway from retina which bypasses the V1/V2 and relaying through the pulvinar of thalamus, reaches area V5. Hence, perception of movement may sometimes be possible even in absence of vision (blind sight). Damage to area V5 leads to akinetopsia. Such a person would be able to identify a bird when it is sitting on a tree, but not when it is flying in the sky. On the other hand, area V5 is developed quite early after birth (after V1/V2 which are developed before birth) as babies find movement very interesting. The area V5 has a two-way connection with the area V1/V2 through which connection is established with other cortical areas which might include the frontal cortex. I hypothesize, at this stage, that imagination of movement (as would any type of imaginative thinking does) evokes frontal cortical activation and that would in turn might evoke activation of cells in V5 to appreciate this motion (imaginative). Oriented lines when set in motion stimulate V5 most. Hence, lines drawn in different orientation on a painting to depict motion may be assumed to stimulate V5 neurons incorporating frontal cortical activation evoking an imaginative sensation of movement. We shall come back to this concept when we discuss dynamism in a static art form. In addition to its intimate connection with area V1/V2, area V5 is also intimately connected to area V3 which appreciates shape, size, and form of the object of vision. While this connection is needed for object identification when in motion (for example, a flying bird), this connection, I believe, is exploited by animation film makers. In animation or cartoon films, the same object, in changed shapes, is presented in rapid sequence to the visual cortex especially area V3 for appreciation of shape and form. When done rapidly, the sensation activates area V5 (through V3) giving the illusion of movement.

PRINCIPLES OF ART SCIENCE

Ramachandran and Hirstein,[3] in their seminal article, described nine principles of art science or the science of aesthetics, as they called it. As all these principles are based on functioning of the human brain and especially the visual brain, I would prefer to call these the principles of art neuroscience or neuroaesthetics. I shall only briefly mention the first three major principles here and mention their relationship to brain function. The "peak-shaft principle" which allows an artist to depict the essence of a topic by exaggerating the details (for example, Picasso's Cubist phase paintings of exaggerating the breasts and hips) really signifies brain's quest for the essentials. "Grouping or binding principle", in which the artist binds together multiple bits into a coherent whole (for example, Henri Matisse's paintings), really portrays the grouping or binding function of the visual brain. Lastly, the "visual isolation principle" is an artistic principle by which an artist uses just a few lines to capture and express the essence of a visual concept (for example, Picasso's Dove series) really evokes imaginative thinking which involves frontal cortical activation.

DYNAMISM: A NEW PRINCIPLE OF ART NEUROSCIENCE

At this stage, I introduce the concept for existence of a new principle which I wish to call "dynamism". What is dynamism in a visual scene and how does it contribute to visual aesthetics? I would like the reader to imagine two visual scenes:

Firstly, imagine yourself sitting on the beach in a clear sunny day, the wind is blowing mildly, the sea is quiet—not much breakers and the boats are sailing smoothly. Compare this scene with a second one. Imagine yourself sitting on a beach on a cloudy day, the wind is strong, the sea is rough, there are high waves and tall white foamy breakers with a roaring sound and the little boats at a distance tossing and tumbling. Which scene would appeal to you more? Most people told me of the second scene where there was much movement. This is dynamism in a visual scene and it appeals to most as there is strong stimulation of the visual area V5/MT, as we appreciate the motion. The same principle applies to visual and other forms of art. A movie or a video is generally more appreciative than a still photograph. An orchestra where there is much fluctuation of volume (like the Bolero by Maurice Ravel) is often more appreciative than a "placid" one (like the Pavane Pour Une Infante Defunte by the same composer). But what about painting/sculpture which is fundamentally a static image?

An object of art like a painting becomes more appreciative when it activates more and more number of cortical neurons in the brain (mostly visual brain) and more and more cortical areas (visual or otherwise).[2] A painting/sculpture generally evokes aesthetic experience through activation of areas V1/V2, V3, and V4. If V5/MT, the motion area, can also be activated (truly as in a movie or through imaginative frontal activation as discussed earlier), the aesthetic value or appreciativeness of the art form can be enhanced. Paintings and sculptures of dancing human figures are thus more appreciative than static (sitting or standing) ones. Compare **Figures 2 and 3**—both bronze sculptures of Hindu deities. The feminine one (Goddess Saraswati) is certainly more appealing than the male one (Lord Krishna) as the former is in a dancing posture and one can imagine the dancing sequence in a function of time. This is dynamism—appreciation of which is partly through imagination, that is frontal cortical activation and also V5 stimulation. Michelangelo's paintings in the Sistine Chapel are classic examples of such types of "explicit dynamism" where movements are very obvious needing only a little amount of imaginative thinking. Consider the David and Goliath **(Fig. 4)**. As David's sword is held up, the two arms are not in the same plane, the right one is much backward (one gets a three-dimensional realization) and the position of the right arm must be changing with time as the sward would come down to Goliath's head. So, one imagines a four-dimensional (time factor included) scene. This is what explicit dynamism does to an apparently static visual scene (like a painting). Through depiction of dynamism, the art watcher gets a 3D realization of a 2D canvas and then to a 4D imagination of the entire visual scene. The artist does this by employing techniques through which he can evoke imaginative frontal lobar activation and area V5/MT stimulation. Dynamism, thus, increases the aesthetic value of an art work by stimulating more and more cerebral cortical neurons and areas—visual or otherwise.

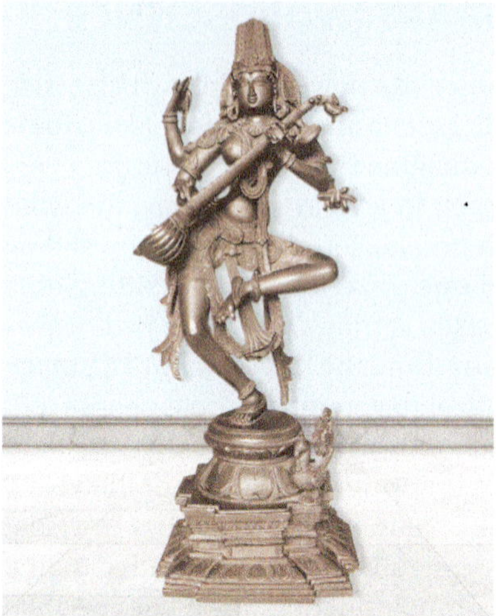

FIG. 2: Goddess Saraswati.

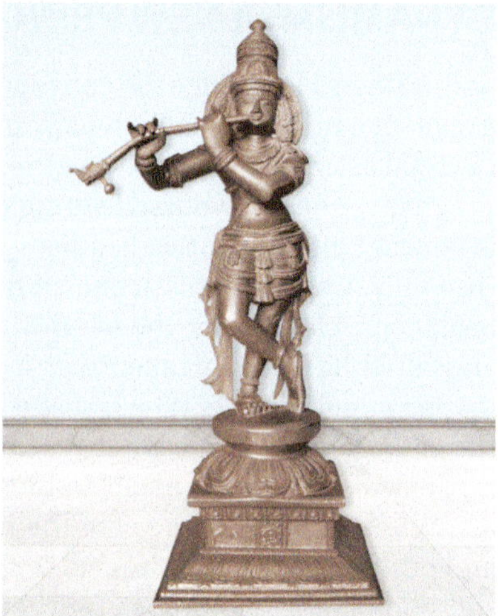

FIG. 3: Lord Krishna.

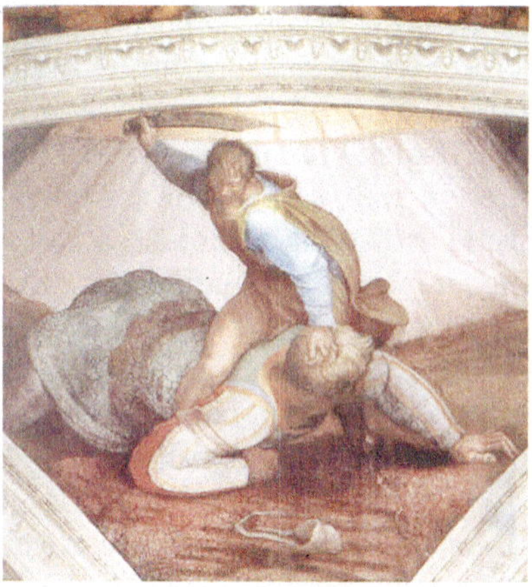

FIG. 4: Explicit dynamism: David and Goliath (Michelangelo—Sistine Chapel).

I would now try to draw the attention of readers to a somewhat different form of dynamism where imaginative thinking is more than what exactly is depicted by the artist in reality. The artist, of course, very intelligently applies this technique and exploits brain function of imaginative thinking with frontal lobar activation and some activation of V5. I shall call this "implicit dynamism" as opposed to "explicit dynamism" as discussed earlier. **Figures 5A and B** are paintings of Claude Monet which are displayed side by side (again very intelligently) at the Musée d'Orsay in Paris. Both depict a lady with an umbrella walking through a meadow. Note the change in direction of movement of the lady from **Figures 5A and B**. Consequently, due to changed direction of wind flow in relation to the

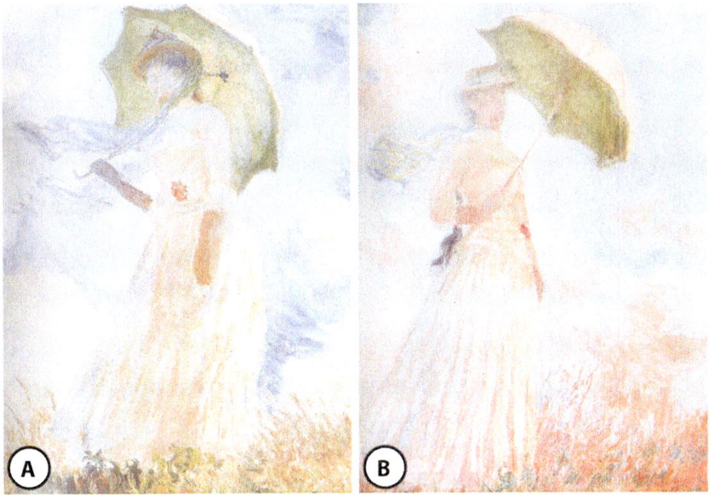

FIGS. 5A AND B: Implicit dynamism (Claude Monet).

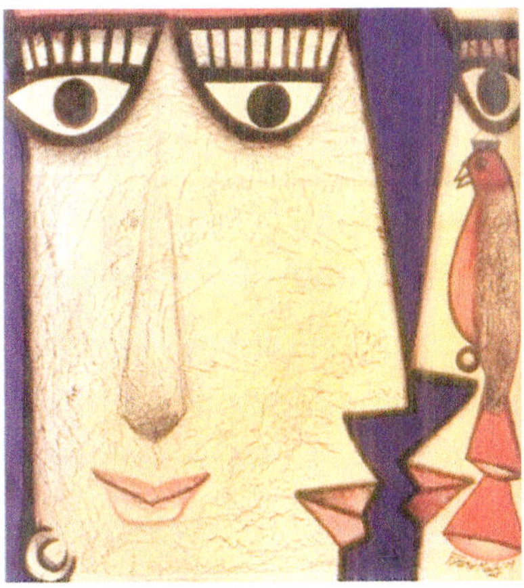

FIG. 6: Implicit dynamism (Paresh Maity).

lady's path of walking, the direction of tilting of the lady's umbrella is different between the two paintings. Also, the lady's scarf seems to be flowing in a different plane as the strong wind flow direction has changed. Monet clearly wanted to highlight this wind flow motion change in these two paired paintings. This is a classic example of what I wish to convey as "implicit dynamism". The same can be observed in other artists' works and fundamentally calls for imaginative thinking and frontal lobar activation on the part of the viewer. An example of implicit dynamism is depicted in **Figure 6** by Paresh Maity. Herein a lady looking straight ahead, the artist gives an impression in the same painting as the lady turns her head to the left to speak to her friend. It is a classic example of implicit dynamism.

KINETIC ART AND DYNAMISM

Zeki and Lamb[4] introduced the concept of kinetic art which according to them "represents a reductionist approach which emphasizes motion and deemphasizes both form and color or at least renders them insignificant." Basically, in kinetic art, objective motion plays a dominant part or the perception of motion is strongly induced by a static figure. This, according to the authors, primarily occurs through V5/MT stimulation and they remain silent on the issue of imaginative thinking through frontal lobar activation. The concept of kinetic art may have some semblance to what I described as explicit dynamism but this is vastly different from what has been described here as "implicit dynamism". I feel aesthetic experience of an art work cannot be solely determined by laying emphasis on motion (V5 activation) but is contributed by color and form of the art work (V4 and V3 activation) as also, the imaginative element (frontal cortex). I, therefore, feel that what I describe here as dynamism in art is exactly not the same as what had been described earlier as kinetic art.

CONCLUDING REMARKS

Why is Mona Lisa smiling: The final hypothesis

As mentioned earlier, Gombrich[1] opined that Leonardo very intelligently painted Mona Lisa's angles of the mouth to depict her smile. I would, at the end, go a step forward to suggest that the painter actually did it very intelligently to introduce an element of implicit dynamism, an imagination of movement of a smiling face, in the painting to increase the aesthetic value of his art work. I suggest that a photographer employs the same technique when he asks his subjects to say "cheese" as he wishes to introduce an element of dynamism in his art work (namely photograph) to increase its appreciativeness or aesthetic value. A smile is only a transient phenomenon, it cannot be permanent, but the enigma left on Mona Lisa's smiling face seems to have left a permanent effect on the viewers for centuries. Leonardo did have a profound knowledge of human anatomy but the existence of area V5/MT had been described centuries later. It seems Mona Lisa has really something to smile about now that the puzzle appears to have been solved!

REFERENCES

1. Gombrich EH. The Story of Art. London: Phaidon Press; 1995.
2. Zeki S. Inner Vision. Oxford: Oxford University Press; 1999.
3. Ramachandran VS, Hirstein W. The science of Art. A neurological theory of aesthetic experience. J Consc Stud. 1999;6:15-51.
4. Zeki S, Lamb M. The neurology of kinetic art. Brain. 1994;117:607-36.

(Reproduced with modification from: Chakravarty A. Medical Hypothesis 2010;75:69-72)

CHAPTER

5

Neural Circuitry of Visual Artistic Production and Appreciation: A Proposition

INTRODUCTION

In this essay, the author would like to hypothesize on the likely neural circuitry involved in visual artistic production and appreciation. The propositions presented are based on established and previously conceived concepts relating to the cognitive neuroscience of creativity, principles of visual science, principles of functional neuroanatomy, and lastly, the neurology of centers of appreciation of art and beauty.

PROPOSED NEURAL CIRCUITRY OF VISUAL ARTISTIC PRODUCTION: BACKGROUND

Cognitive Neuroscience of Creativity

The concept of creativity, in general, is an abstract one and simply speaking it involves doing something novel that ultimately proves to be good to the human society. Artistry is indeed a creative endeavor as art imparts knowledge and pleasure to the viewer. Many create art or music and, logically, all may be considered creative. What then differentiates a Leonardo or Michelangelo or Mozart from the rest? Nancy Andreasen had written about ordinary versus extraordinary creativity.[1] But, what determines this extraordinary creativity is not exactly known. Andreasen[1] suggests that extraordinary creative people probably have an extra degree of connectivity in their brains or perhaps harbor an unusual type of connectivity. This is difficult to prove as, of all the extraordinary creative individuals that we know of, only Albert Einstein's brain had been subjected to histological studies, but that too in a very limited fashion. Einstein's brain seemed to have an altered white/gray matter ratio,[2] which was later conceived as suggestive of an extra degree of connectivity.[3] Although creativity is likely to be a phenomenon of mind and hence somewhat abstract, it is indeed a brain phenomenon. Patients with brain injuries perform poorly on creativity tasks. But, where then lies the "Seat" of creativity in the brain? We do not know. Arne

Dietrich, in a recent review, has discussed the current thoughts on the cognitive neuroscience of creativity, summarizing the vast literature on functions of individual brain areas and observations made on brain-injured patients.[4] The role of the prefrontal lobe has been much stressed, although it is far from clear whether it can be called the seat of creativity.

Seat of Artistic Creativity

The brain is incredibly elegant but remains very mysterious. There are several areas of the brain that can be associated with the ability to produce art. Because frontal lobes are highly developed in humans compared with nonhuman primates who cannot produce art, it might be reasonable to deduce that art arises from these structures. However, it seems more likely that the posterior parietal lobe, in particular on the nondominant side, is central to the ability to produce art. Visual artistic production involves a high degree of visual spatial skill.

Following McDonald Critchley's observation that lesions in the nondominant posterior parietal lobe or parietooccipital region cause significant visual spatial motor skill derangement,[5] it is reasonable to suggest that this region of the brain is ultimately associated with artistic production. It has been known for over a century that injuries to the right posterior parietal lobe cause loss of artistic ability. This decline in ability had been detailed in a patient who suffered a series of strokes.[6] Furthermore, visuospatial function has been localized in the nondominant inferior parietal lobe by neuroimaging studies.

On the other hand, some patients with predominantly left brain lesions (frontotemporal dementias and autism) may show unmasking of artistic creativity stored in the right parietal lobe.[7] This somewhat paradoxical observation can be explained on the basis of the theory of "paradoxical functional facilitation" proposed by Kapur.[8] This is thought to occur as a compensatory augmentation occurring as a specific manifestation of central nervous system plasticity. The present author had referred to this earlier as reverse diaschisis.[9] In diaschisis, as first described by von Monakow in 1914, reduced function of one brain area leads to reduced function of a remote brain area to which it is anatomically connected. The reverse occurs here. The localization of artistic creativity in the right intraparietal sulcal region has been further suggested by the report, by Seeley et al.,[10] of a patient with primary progressive aphasia (due to corticobasal degeneration) who showed unusual transmodal creativity (auditory to visual). The lady had a fairly circumscribed atrophy of her left inferior frontal-anterior temporal cortex, but seemed to have an excess of gray matter in the right intraparietal sulcal region. This lady, on being fascinated by Maurice Ravel's composition of Bolero, painted the "music" beautifully in an art form. And, this phenomenon of development of *de novo* creativity is not just limited in the field of visual art but had been observed in fields of music and literature as well.[11] On the other hand, this hemispheric model is undoubtedly a simplification. Lythgoe et al.[12] reported on a patient who, in contrast to frontotemporal dementia patients, developed a prolific visual artistic output in the context of a preserved language function that also enabled a prolific written poetic output. The subject had bilateral middle cerebral artery aneurysms.

Conversely, Drago et al.[13] reported in an artist with Parkinson's disease whose artistic qualities significantly deteriorated following left subthalamic nucleus (STN) deep brain stimulation (DBS), suggesting the role of the dominant hemisphere in art production that may be more than simply a deficit of motor executive function. The problem certainly is more complex in patients with bihemispheric dysfunction. The contribution of both hemispheres in creative cognition is exemplified in split-brain subjects with incomplete surgical division of corpus callosum as suggested by the lack of creativity in these subjects[14] probably because they cannot transmit nonverbal or emotive signals from one hemisphere to the other.[15] These studies, however, do not definitely suggest that the "seat" of artistic creativity is in the right inferior parietal lobe, but can only point to the significant role that this area plays in visual artistic production.

Role of Prefrontal Lobe in Creativity

Arne Dietrich summarized the vast amount of literature that exists in relation to functions of the prefrontal lobe, especially those related to creativity.[4] However, again, it is far from clear that this too can be called the "seat" of any creative process. The prefrontal lobes, however, control imaginative thinking and the final expression of emotion—functions needed in visual artistic appreciation (to be discussed later). The prefrontal lobe can be considered to have two distinct parts—the ventromedial prefrontal lobe (VMPFL) and the dorsolateral prefrontal lobe (DLPFL). These two parts are phylogenetically different—the VMPFL is developed from hippocampal tissue and does not possess any extensive cortical connectivity except perhaps with the anterior temporal lobe structures through the uncinate fasciculus (UF) (vide infra). It has been suggested that the process of creative cognition (including artistic creative conceptualization) starts at the VMPFL and is then transferred to the DLPFL, which, because of its wide connectivity, activates other necessary cortical areas (in both hemispheres) to determine the final creative output. Visual artistic production would be no exception.

Concept of Two Visual Systems

Ungerleider and Mishikin[16] and later Goodale and Westwood[17] conceived of the existence of two cortical visual systems. The ventral stream connects the occipital with the anterior temporal lobe and is called the "what" system. The dorsal stream connects the occipital lobe to the frontal and parietal cortices, and can be called the "where" system. For example, if one views a car, the image is formed in the visual cortex on the occipital lobe. This information is transmitted through the ventral stream to the anterior temporal lobe where the perceived image is matched with the stored memory in the hippocampal region, and one identifies the object of vision as a "car." But, where is the car? Transfer of information from the occipital to the parietal lobe through the dorsal stream would tell one where exactly is the car—in the garage or in the street. These two visual systems are intimately involved in both visual artistic production and appreciation or painting meaningful art. This has been demonstrated in disorders involving these visual pathways (e.g., semantic dementia[18] and Balint syndrome[19]). With semantic dementia, it is possible to generate beautiful paintings with the more posterior portion of the brain without being able to ascribe a meaning onto what has been painted. For example, a patient can draw a bird, but lack the formal word knowledge about how a bird differs from another animal.[18] Smith and his colleagues[19] described a patient in whom temporary dysfunction in the dorsal stream led an artist to simplify visually rich paintings into paintings that captured only small pieces of an object. When her vision returned, the full internally generated pictures returned. But, what are the gross neuroanatomical equivalents of these conceptual systems?

Neuroanatomical Correlates of Two Visual Systems

Different cortical areas in each cerebral hemisphere are interconnected with each other through a series of well-defined and dissectible bundles of white fibers **(Fig. 1)**. The arcuate fibers are curved bundles that connect adjacent cortical areas. The superior longitudinal fasciculus (SLF) connects the occipital lobe with the parietal and frontal cortices curving over the corpus callosum. The inferior longitudinal fasciculus (ILF) connects the occipital lobe to the anterior temporal lobar structures, including the hippocampo-amygdaloid complex. The SLF can be considered to be the gross anatomical counterpart of the "dorsal stream," and the ILF as the anatomical counterpart of the "ventral stream" of the two visual systems concept detailed earlier. There is yet another major white fiber tract not much discussed in the cognitive/visual neuroscience literature. This is the UF that loops round the Sylvian fissure and connects the anterior temporal lobar structures to the frontal cortex. As would be detailed later, this fasciculus is likely to be intimately connected with artistic activity as it connects the emotional and memory brain to the frontal lobe, especially the VMPFL. Of course, emotions are mostly mediated through the Papez circuit of the limbic system connects the amygdala and the hippocampus through the fornicial system to the mammillary bodies and then on to the anterior nucleus of thalamus and further on to the frontal cortex to determine the final expression of the emotion.

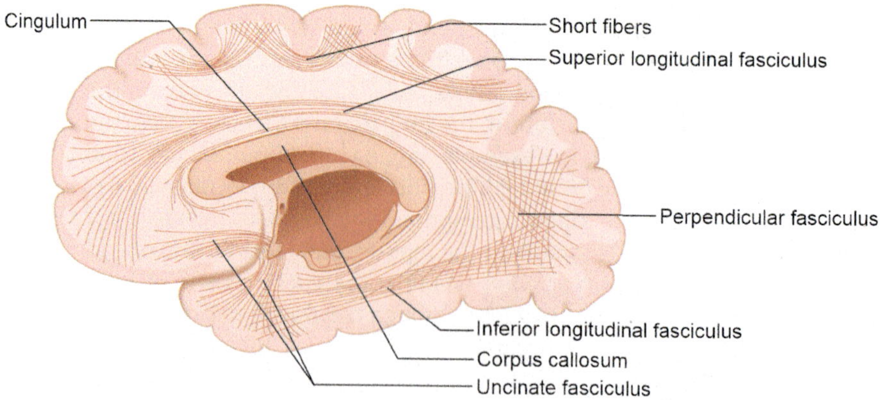

FIG. 1: Major white matter interconnecting tracts in the cerebrum.

Source: Adapted from Williams PL. Gray' Anatomy, 38th edition. Edinburgh: Churchill Livingstone; 1995.

Based on these established and long-conceived neuroanatomical pathways, cognitive neuroscientific principles, and principles of visual science and systems, I would now proceed to speculate on the neural pathways (circuitry) of both visual artistic production and appreciation.

PROPOSED NEURAL CIRCUITRY FOR VISUAL ARTISTIC PRODUCTION

The present author's hypothetical neural circuitry for visual artistic production is shown schematically in **Figure 2**.

The author suggests that when an artist conceptualizes a visual scene that he wishes to paint or sculpture, activation first occurs in the VMPFL, which, as discussed earlier, is the site of origin of creative cognition. This activation, which results in the cognition of the visual image, is influenced by inputs to the VMPFL from the memory brain (memory of witnessing similar situation in the past) in the hippocampal region of anterior temporal lobe through the UF. The VMPFL activity is also influenced by the emotion of the artist in relation to the perceived concept of the visual scene, carried from the emotional brain (amygdalo-hippocampal complex also in anterior temporal lobe) through the fornicial system of fibers constituting the limbic system pathway (Papez circuit).

Once the concept of the art to be created informed in the VMPFL, information is transferred to the DLPFL through the arcuate association fibers for the executive planning of the artwork. The DLFPL performs this by transferring the concept to the visual brain in the occipital lobe (through the SLF or dorsal stream of visual system) to form the visual image to be painted. Bidirectional impulse transmission through the SLF allows constant modification of the visual image of

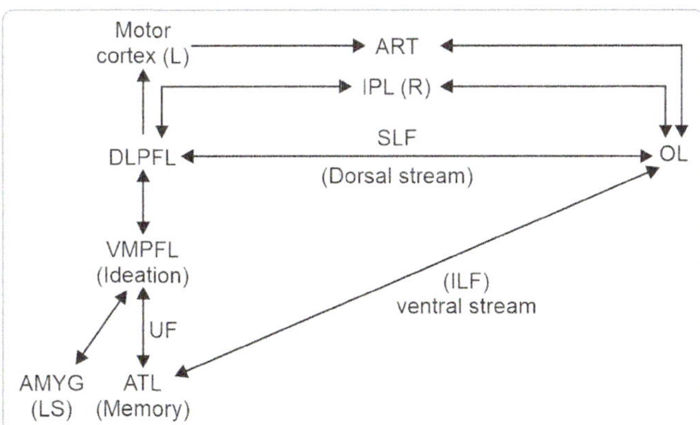

FIG. 2: Schematic diagram showing hypothesized neural circuitry for visual artistic production.

(DLPFL: dorsolateral prefrontal lobe; VMPFL: ventromedial prefrontal lobe; IPL: inferior parietal lobule; SLF: superior longitudinal fasciculus; ILF: inferior longitudinal fasciculus; ATL: anterior temporal lobe; UF: uncinate fasciculus; AMYG: Amygdala; LS: limbic system; OL: occipital lobe)

the concept till it is finalized. This process is also influenced by feedback from the anterior temporal lobar structures (memory and emotional brain) to the occipital lobe through the ILF (the ventral stream of visual system). The information regarding the concept of the artwork, as also of the visual image being formed, traverses to the inferior parietal lobule (IPL) (the storehouse of artistic creativity) as the SLF relays through the parietal cortex on its passage while connecting the frontal and occipital cortices.

The IPL gives artistic coloring to the visual image till the final form is reached. Once the final form of the visual image to be painted or sculptured is formed, the information is finally "handed over" to the DLPFL through bidirectional pathway in the SLF. The DLPFL, being well connected to the other areas in the frontal and parietal lobe, transfers the information to the motor cortex for final execution of the artwork—the artist puts the brush and paint on the canvas or the chisel and hammer on a piece of stone. As the artwork is being formed, it is constantly viewed by the visual brain (occipital lobe) and information is sent and exchanged with the artistic creativity area in the IPL and the memory and emotional brains in the anterior temporal lobe through the bidirectional network in SLF and ILF. Modifications perceived are finally transferred to the DLPFL for final execution. It is suggested that the process in essence is not a stepwise one as escribed but works in unison and is not rested till the final artwork is completed.

PROPOSED NEURAL CIRCUITRY FOR VISUAL ARTISTIC APPRECIATION

Background

The neurology of artistic appreciation (visual or otherwise) is an utterly complex process. This involves principles of neuroaesthetics, a new subspecialty of neurosciences. The subject had been exhaustively discussed in a recent monograph.[20]

The author does not wish to go into the details of neuroaesthetic principles but would simply like to highlight the brain areas that are implicated in aesthetic experience of visual art. In fact, technically, it is easier to map brain areas (by functional MRI technology) involved in art appreciation than locating areas concerned in artistic production—as artists cannot be asked to create art while lying inside a MRI gantry but a subject can surely look at and appreciate a piece of art projected before his eyes through a mirror system in the gantry.

Chatterjee[21] suggested that the involvement of the visual brain region in processing aesthetic stimuli is the same as in the processing of any other kind of visual stimuli. What sets aesthetic preference apart from other cognitive processes involving visual stimuli is precisely the engagement of additional nonperceptual processes such as emotions and decision making.

These nonperceptual processes ultimately evoke the feeling of appreciation (the "Ah" experience) or perhaps feeling of rejection in the mind of the viewer. Recent neuroimaging studies have revealed a basic picture of the neural correlates of these cognitive and affective processes. Affective processes involved in aesthetic appreciation seem to be mediated by the orbitofrontal (or ventromedial prefrontal—VMPFL) cortex,[22] caudate nucleus, anterior cingulated cortex, and strengthening of early visual processes in the occipital cortex.[23] Recognition and meaning attribution in aesthetic appreciation seem to be related with activity in the temporal pole,[24] and decisions seemed to be mediated by the lateral prefrontal cortex (DLPFL) and the frontal pole.[24,25] The prefrontal lobe thus appears to be pivotal in art appreciation, just like as discussed before, in art production.

Activity in the orbitofrontal or ventromedial prefrontal cortex was identified by Kawabata and Zeki[22] while participants decided (decision making function as mentioned earlier) about the beauty of diverse artistic visual stimuli. The fact that many studies have observed activity in this region in association with primary and abstract rewarding stimuli suggests that its role in aesthetic preference might be to represent the reward value of each visual stimulus. On the other hand, studies carried out by Cela-Conde et al.[25] and Jacobsen et al.[24] revealed that rating the beauty of visual artworks and geometric designs engages the lateral prefrontal cortex (DLPFL).

PROPOSED NEURAL CIRCUITRY FOR VISUAL ARTISTIC APPRECIATION

The author would now proceed to hypothesize on the neural circuitry involved in artistic appreciation in a somewhat stepwise manner **(Fig. 3)**, although the author believes that the entire circuitry is activated simultaneously and not exactly in a stepwise manner (described here only to put a complex concept in a simple and easily understandable fashion).

When an artwork is viewed, the image is formed in the visual brain. Many visual areas in the occipital lobe are activated to appreciate the shape, size, form, and color of the artwork.

Activation of the fusiform gyrus would occur if familiar faces or buildings are visualized and would evoke a different kind of emotion.

The visual image from the occipital lobe is then transferred both to the frontal and to the parietal lobes (through the dorsal stream or SLF—the "where"

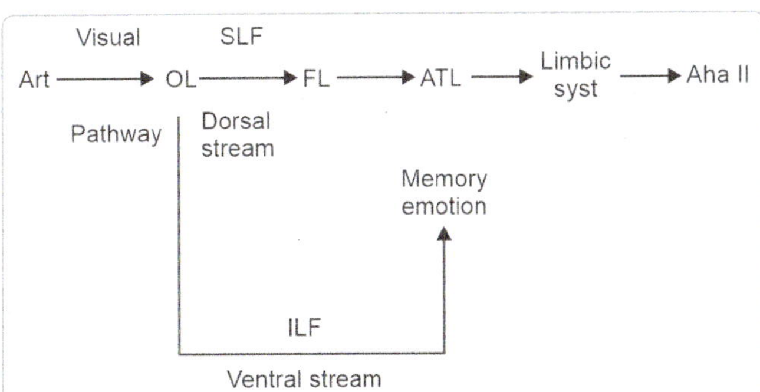

FIG. 3: Schematic diagram showing hypothesized neural circuitry for visual artistic appreciation. (FL: frontal lobe; ILF: inferior longitudinal fasciculus; ATL: anterior temporal lobe; OL: occipital lobe)

system) as also to the anterior temporal lobe (through the ventral stream or ILF—the "what" system). At the anterior temporal lobe, activation leads to evoking memory and emotion. These are then transferred to the frontal lobe (both VMPFL and DLPFL) for appreciation of beauty as also for imaginative thinking, and may evoke a "conflict".

Information relating to the final result of this integration at the prefrontal lobar level is finally again transferred back to the emotional brain (amygdalo-hippocampal complex) in the anterior temporal lobe through the UF. The final result is activation of the limbic system through the Papez circuit and the "Ah" experience.

FURTHER THOUGHTS

Two other functions in relation to artistic appreciation may be ascribed to the prefrontal cortex. Firstly, this is the site of imaginative thinking and hence must be activated when subjects view unfinished artworks and imagine how the artwork would have looked if finished (e.g., many of the sculptures by Michelangelo) and also to appreciate elements of movement or dynamism in a static art form as discussed by the present author earlier.[26] Imaginative thinking on the part of the viewer is also involved in appreciation of both abstract and symbolic arts.

Secondly, the prefrontal cortex is also engaged in the phenomenon of "frontal lobar conflict" when an artwork viewed is "mentally" compared with similar images and visual scenes previously perceived and stored in the memory brain of the anterior temporal lobe. The information from the latter area is transferred to the prefrontal lobe through the UF as had been conceived earlier in this article. This gives rise to heightened activation in the prefrontal lobe, which, then being transferred to the anterior temporal lobe again through the UF, activates the limbic system to evoke emotion of appreciation (the "Ah" experience). Support for this hypothesis comes from the work of Zeki and colleagues,[27] who showed, by functional neuroimaging, that there occurs greater frontal lobar activation when subjects viewed objects dressed in unnatural colors than in their usual ones. The reason, of course, is the conflict between the perceived image and the image stored in memory from previous experience. The phenomenon obviously comes into play when subjects appreciate innovations made by the artist, e.g., in impressionist art forms.

CONCLUDING REMARKS

So far, our present day concepts of the brain areas involved in either artistic production or appreciation of art and beauty are based on observational studies made in patients (often artists) where the diseased part of the brain could be localized with reasonable accuracy using sophisticated neuroimaging means or subjecting control subjects with various visual stimuli (e.g., beautiful artworks) presented before their eyes using a mirror from a TV screen as they lie in a functional MRI or positron emission tomography scan gantry. Such techniques, although useful, seem to be very basic in relation to the complexity of the subject under study. What is needed is actually to study the brains of artists as they work or a common man as he stands before a masterpiece. Currently available technologies are far from achieving these targets. Perhaps, someday, we may hope to have functional MRI/positron emission tomography done by more refined machines with wider gantry when it would be possible to actually visualize brain area activation in artists engaged in painting or a common man enjoying a beautiful artwork. What had been hypothesized here regarding the possible neural circuitry for artistic production and appreciation is a very simplistic version of an utterly complex process. The proposed hypotheses are entirely conceptual needing experimental proof through available and yet to develop more sophisticated neuroimaging and electrophysiological techniques. However, the hypotheses are indeed based on established principles of neuroanatomy, cognitive neurosciences, and deductions from described case studies in cognitive neurology. The author would stress again that nothing in reality occurs in a stepwise fashion, the whole circuitry involved is activated simultaneously and continues to remain so long after an artist creates an art or a viewer views a masterpiece. "Art is the expression of the inner world of an artist." It is highly unlikely that principles of gross anatomy would ever be able to decipher the mysteries of this "inner world."

REFERENCES

1. Andreasen N. The Creative Brain. The Science of genius. London: PLUME (Penguin Group); 2005.
2. Diamond MC, Schiebel AB, Murphy JG, Hervey T. On the brain of a scientist: Albert Einstein. Exp Neurol. 1985;88:198-204.
3. Heilman KM, Nadeau SE, Beversdorf DU. Creative innovation: Possible brain mechanisms. Neurocase. 2003;9:369-79.
4. Dietrich A. The cognitive neuroscience of creativity. Psychon Bull Rev. 2004;11:1011-26.
5. Critchley M. The parietal lobes. New York: Hafner Publications; 1953.
6. Miller BL. Creativity in the context of neurologic illness. CNS Spectr. 2008;13:7-9.
7. Pollak TA, Mulvenne CM, Lythgoe NF. De novo artistic behaviour following brain injury. In: Bogousslavsky J, Hennerici MG (Eds). Neurological Disorders in Famous Artists—Part 2. Basel: Karger; 2007. pp. 75-88.
8. Kapur N. Paradoxical functional facilitation in brain-behaviour research. A critical review. Brain. 1996;119:1775-90.
9. Chakravarty A. The creative brain – Revisiting concepts. Med Hypotheses. 2010;74:606-12.
10. Seeley WW, Mathews BR, Richard K, Gorno-Tempini MC, Foti D, Mackenzie IR, et al. Unravelling Bolero: Progressive aphasia, transmodal creativity and the right posterior neocortex. Brain. 2008;131:39-49.
11. Miller BL, Boone K, Cummings JL, Read SL, Mishkin F. Functional correlates of musical and visual ability in frontotemporal dementia. Br J Psychiatry. 2001;76:458-63.
12. Lythgoe MF, Pollak TA, Kalmus M, De Haan M, Chong WK. Obsessive, prolific artistic output following subarachnoid hemorrhage. Neurology. 2005;64:397-8.
13. Drago V, Foster PS, Okun MS, Cosentino FI, Conigliaro R, Haq I, et al. Turning off artistic ability: The influence of left DBS in art production. J Neurol Sci. 2008;281:116-21.
14. Gazzaniga MS. Consciousness and the cerebral hemisphere. In: Gazzaniga MS (Ed). The Cognitive Neurosciences. Cambridge, Massachusetts: MIT Press; 1995. pp. 1391-404.
15. Bogan JE, Bogan GM. Creativity and the corpus callosum. Psych Clin N Am. 1988;11:293-301.
16. Ungerleider LG, Mishikin M. Two cortical visual systems. In: Ingle DJ, Goodale MA, Mansdold RJ (Eds). The Analysis of Visual Behavior. Cambridge, Massachusetts: MIT Press; 1982. pp. 549-66.

17. Goodale MA, Westwood DA. An evolving view of duplex vision: Separate but interacting cortical pathways for perception and action. Curr Opin Neurobiol. 2004;14:203-11.
18. Miller BL. Hou CF. Portraits of artists: Emergence of visual creativity in dementia. Arch Neurol. 2004;61:842-4.
19. Smith WS, Mindelzun RE, Miller BL. Simultanagnosia through the eyes of an artist. Neurology. 2003;60:1832-4.
20. Skov M, Vartanian O. Neuroaesthetics. New York: Baywood Publishing Company Inc.; 2009.
21. Chatterjee A. Prospects for a cognitive neuroscience of visual aesthetics. Bull Psychol Arts. 2003;4:55-60.
22. Kawabata H, Zeki S. Neural correlates of beauty. J Neurophysiol. 2004;91:1699-705.
23. Vartanian O, Goel V. Neuroanatomical correlates of aesthetic preference for paintings. Neuroreport. 2004;15:893-7.
24. Jacobsen T, Schubotz RI, Hofel L, Von Cramon DY. Brain correlates of aesthetic judgement of beauty. Neuroimage. 2005;29:276-85.
25. Cela-Conde CJ, Marty G, Maestu F, Ortiz T, Munar E, Fernandez A, et al. Activation of prefrontal cortex in the human visual aesthetic perception. Proc Natl Acad Sci USA. 2004;101:6321-5.
26. Chakravarty A. Mona Lisa's smile: A hypothesis based on a new principle of art neuroscience. Med Hypotheses. 2010;75:69-72.
27. Zeki S, Marini L. Three cortical stages of color processing in the human brain. Brain 1998;121:1669-85.

(Reproduced with modifications from: Chakravarty A. The neural circuitry of visual artistic production and appreciation: A proposition. Ann Indian Acad Neurol. 2012;15(2):71-5.)

CHAPTER

6

Art and Epilepsy as Depicted by Modern and Contemporary Artists with Epilepsy

INTRODUCTION

The term epilepsy (epikgwía) is originated from the Greek word epilambanein (epikalbmeim), which means "to seize, possess, or afflict". Different authors have referred to the condition over the years with different meanings namely a disease of the moon, sacred disease, and demonism.[1] Babylonians and Egyptians recognized seizures as being associated with physical illnesses like head injury, but, like the Greeks and Romans, sometimes thought them to be more magical or occult than physical.[2] During the middle ages and the Renaissance, the visual arts in relation to seizures were dominated by religious motifs. The middle ages witnessed an explosion in cults devoted to all kinds of saints.[3] Although the 15th to 20th centuries arts in Europe seemed to be dominated by a rather religious attitude toward epilepsy, the details of seizure semiology often had been quite accurate in the artworks. The history of "the falling sickness" not only reveals much about the culture and artistic trends of the times but also about the state of medical knowledge at that stage.[4] Epilepsy had been of great interests to artists over centuries, and was beautifully displayed in paintings, drawings, sketches, copper engravings, woodcuts, canvases, ceiling frescos, ceramics, sculptures, crafts, and printmaking. "*Epilepsy like art is a reflection of the human condition, and the historical relationship between the two is riveting. In candid form, art reveals much about societal attitudes toward epilepsy and people with epilepsy; it brandishes all that society holds dear—its truths, both beautiful and hideous, its misconceptions, and its emotional thralls.*[4]" In this chapter, the author would review selected paintings done in modern and contemporary periods by artists with epilepsy depicting the various facets of this common disease—once considered a divine illness.[5]

MODERN ARTWORKS

Poor Miss Finch

In the novel "Poor Miss Finch" written by the English author Wilkie Collins,[6] the post-traumatic seizures of a young man (named Oscar) constitute the central

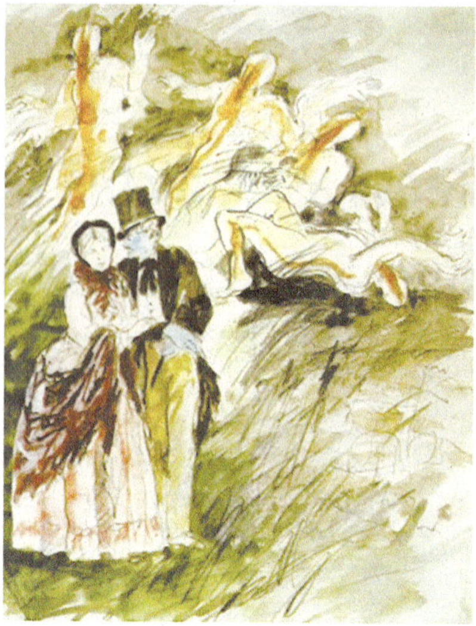

FIG. 1: Poor Miss Finch by unknown artist, 1872, from the book Poor Miss Finch.

theme of the story. Collins provided a very accurate description of a right focal onset versive seizure with secondary generalization in the man which was successfully treated with silver nitrate. This therapy, however, caused discoloration of his skin to blackish blue.[7] Oscar loved the beautiful, but blind Lucilla who also exhibited sudden and unaccountable changes of mood. Lucilla returned Oscar's affections. An ophthalmologist later operated on Lucilla and successfully restored her vision. When blind, Lucilla had a hallucination of a world full of colors, loving everything bright and disliking everything dark. The painting below shows the engaged couple. The different phases of Oscar's generalized tonic–clonic seizures are depicted in the background. The "drama" of the fall during the convulsion is depicted in different stages, from the body standing up straight to it lying on the ground **(Fig. 1)**.[7]

The Red Curtain

The painting below is the symbol of the Stiftung Michael foundation against epilepsy, in Hamburg, Germany. An anonymous artist with epilepsy, assisting in a painting therapy group, painted this around 1965. The painting symbolizes the expression of human hopelessness portraying Vincent Van Gogh who was probably afflicted with epilepsy.[4,6] In the painting, Van Gogh is found lying on the ground; his right leg extended in a tonic posture, while his left leg and both arms are flexed. His eyes are open wide, and the head is turned to the right. The painting depicts an epileptic seizure in a very accurate way with a focus in the left hemisphere probably in the supplementary motor cortex. The knocked-over chair beside Van Gogh probably resulted from the sudden fall of the epileptic spell. The painting has a predominantly red background which probably stands for aggression, power, and evil. The black birds seen through the window might

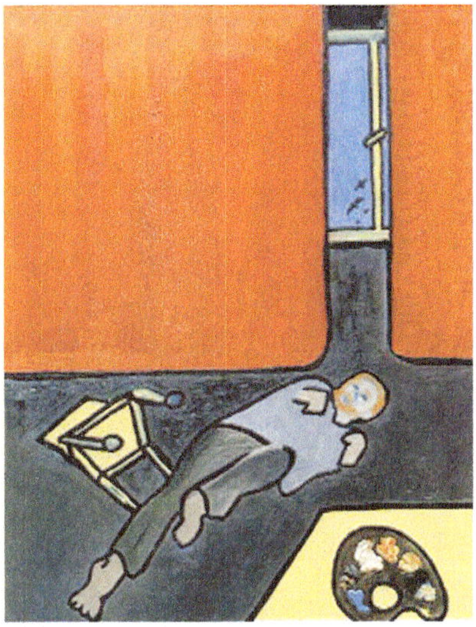

FIG. 2: The red curtain or homage to Vincent, anonymous painter, approximately 1965, German Epilepsy Museum, Kork, Germany.

symbolize the plague and disease-bringing evil spirits. The oil palette lies untouched, representing how epilepsy can jeopardize a person's professional life **(Fig. 2)**.

CONTEMPORARY ARTWORK

Epilepsy, Leaving the Nightmare Behind

The painting below **(Fig. 3)** is a contemporary artwork on epilepsy from Canada.[8] The patient is seen lying on the floor, having an epileptic seizure. Upon recovery (painted in stages), he is found standing erect with the help of his physicians. The painting depicts a good outcome from epilepsy surgery. An assembly of white neurons (signifying health) is painted above the patient's head. A physician holds in his hand a "grid" often used for marking the epileptiform zone during surgery. There is also a pane of glass on the right side that represents the screen used to read the epileptic activity mapped with the grid (electroencephalogram). The golden point lies between the patient and the doctors which is an area to which the viewer's eye is naturally directed. Here, it is represented by the tiger lily—the provincial flower of Saskatchewan, Canada.

To the best of the author's knowledge, this is the first artistic depiction that represents positive feelings and hope for patients with epilepsy.

Wired

Iris Hauser is a Canadian artist hailing from British Columbia.[9] Subsequently, she studied and worked at Nova Scotia (1975), Saskatoon (1977–1979), and Germany (1979–1980). Hauser's portraits are generally rich in narrative detailing but also are symbolistic often based on human conditions like epilepsy. The painting below,

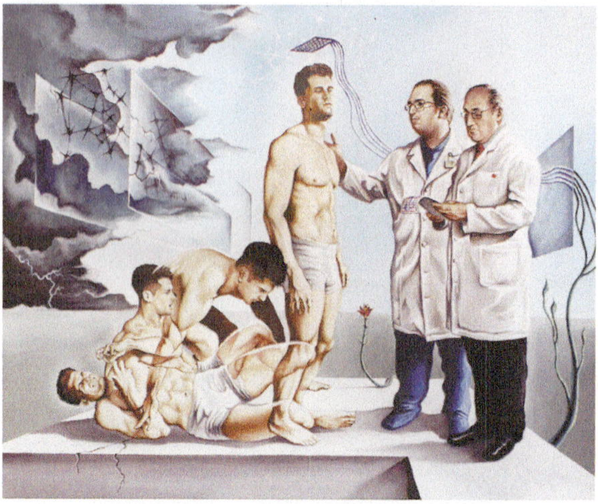

FIG. 3: "Epilepsy, leaving the nightmare behind", 2013. Technique: oil/canvas.

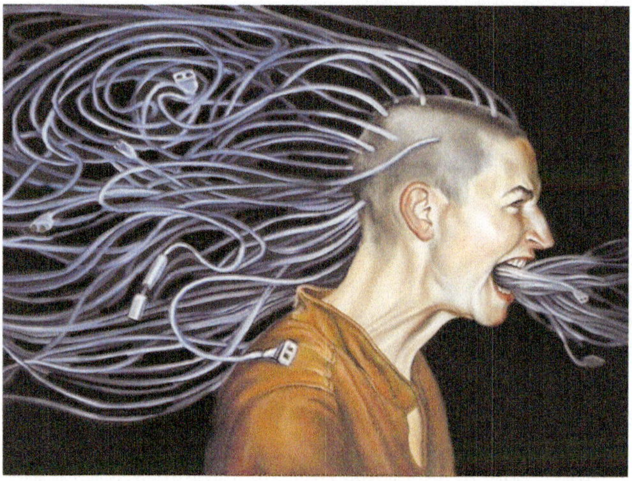

FIG. 4: "Wired", alkyd and oil on canvas 2011, by Iris Hauser, Saskatoon, Saskatchewan, Canada.

titled Wired, was initially symbolistic of frustration originating from operating a computer with hundreds of wired connections in the motherboard. However, there had been ambiguity in the name as also in its interpretations. To be "wired" might mean being emotionally on edge, or it could refer to a connection, as in the wiring of the brain or a reference to neuromodulation. However, the word "wired" might also raise the issue of a modern pathophysiological mechanism of epilepsy—a disease caused by abnormal brain connectivity (abnormal wiring). The subject in the painting represents a patient suffering from problems of connectivity, in the present case, this may be epilepsy **(Fig. 4)**.

Prospective Study in Artists with Epilepsy

Artists with epilepsy often express their views about their disease through their artworks and these provide unique opportunities to acquire knowledge of the experiences of living with epilepsy and associated comorbidities. Steven Sachter tried to provide a glimpse into art collected from a group of artists with epilepsy, focusing on ictal and postictal experiences, psychiatric comorbidities, and social aspects of epilepsy.[10] The collected artworks would go a long way to enhance understanding among doctors of all categories of what it means to have epilepsy as well as to reduce misunderstanding and stigma among the public.

Why would the art created by persons with epilepsy be of interest to healthcare professionals and scientists? First, and perhaps most importantly, the art provides insights into the experience of having seizures (preictal, ictal, and postictal), the psychosocial consequences of living with epilepsy, and the associated comorbidities. Lennox and Markham mentioned over 60 years ago that physicians who treat patients with epilepsy must "match modern drug and surgical therapy with practical sociopsychological therapy" and be "concerned not only with turbulent brain waves but with disturbed emotions..."[1] The treatment of epilepsy in past years focused primarily on controlling seizures; over time, the focus has broadened to include the side effects of therapy, the systemic and psychiatric comorbidities of epilepsy, and the psychosocial consequences of living with epilepsy. Thus, the therapeutic goal has evolved from controlling seizures, at whatever cost, to enabling patients with epilepsy to lead lifestyles that are consistent with their capabilities, ideally free of seizures, medication side effects, and comorbidities.

In Sachter's work, there appear to be four distinct themes in the art: Ictal and postictal experiences as experienced and remembered by the artist, psychiatric comorbidities, social aspects of living with epilepsy, and nonepilepsy related (those problems that have no apparent thematic relationship to epilepsy). The last category is an important reminder that persons with epilepsy, like anyone with a disease diagnosis, should not be judged by their medical condition alone but should rather be appreciated as living human beings and, in the case of the artists, as creative persons, specially gifted to draw and paint.

Much of the art, Sachter had collected, shows the social aspects of living with epilepsy, including feelings of loneliness and isolation from mainstream society **(Fig. 5)** as well as the immediate perceived threat of putting the viewer in the physical position of someone regaining consciousness after having fallen from a seizure, with onlookers both actually and figuratively looking down at the recovering person **(Fig. 6)** and the other revealing the perceived psychological impact of diagnostic technology on one's self-concept **(Fig. 7)**.

CONCLUDING REMARKS

The art created by persons with epilepsy helps us understand what it means to have epilepsy, providing a look into its complexity and comorbidities. On the other hand, the art can bring persons with epilepsy increased understanding

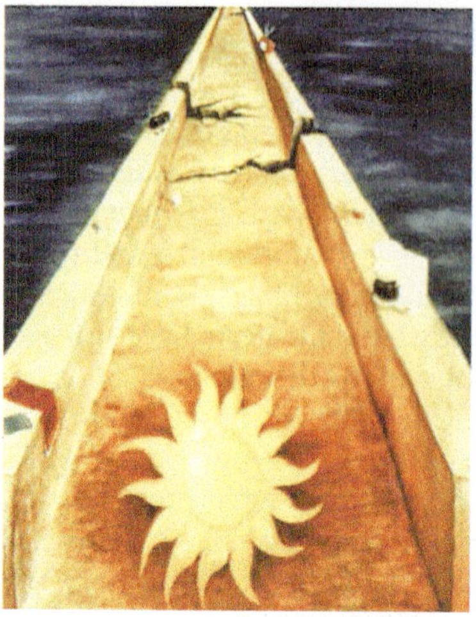

FIG. 5: Interruptions, Wolfgang Fehring.

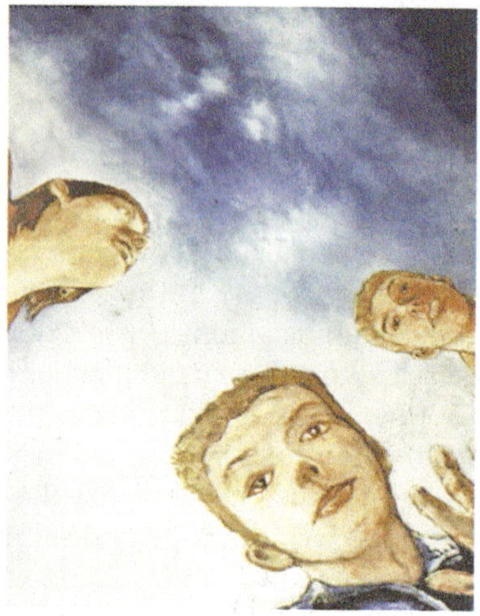

FIG. 6: Faces in circle, Volker Rodermund.

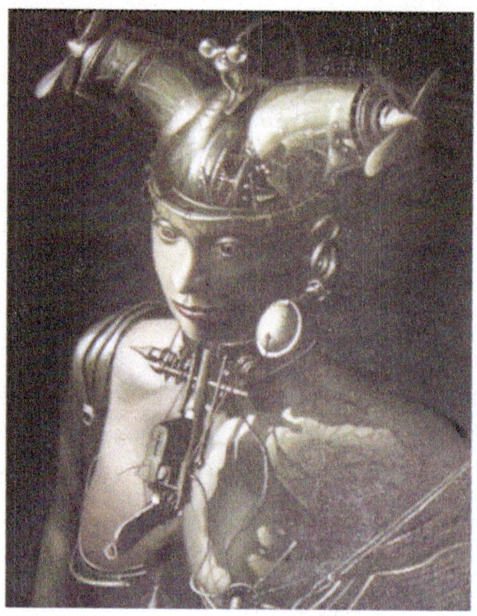

FIG. 7: Ambulatory EEG, Rachna Pettygrove.

and acceptance from clinicians, scientists, and laypersons, especially with regard to their daily experiences and comorbid disorders. It may also be possible to determine whether persons with epilepsy are particularly likely to engage in artistic activities and whether there may be specific characteristics to the art that correlate with side and location of seizure generation.

REFERENCES

1. Magiorkinis E, Sidiropoulou K, Diamantis A. Hallmarks in the history of epilepsy: epilepsy in antiquity. Epilepsy Behav. 2010;17(1):103-8.
2. Fatović-Ferencić S, Dürrigl MA. The sacred disease and its patron saint. Epilepsy Behav. 2001;2(4):370-3.
3. Gross RA. A brief history of epilepsy and its therapy in the Western Hemisphere. Epilepsy Res. 1992;12(2):65-74.
4. Schachter SC. Epilepsy and art. Med J Aust. 1996;164(4):245-8.
5. British Museum, London. Epilepticus sic curabitur. [online] Available from http://www.epilepsiemuseum.de/english/kunst/sicepilepticus.html. [Last accessed January, 2025]
6. Malcolm SJ. Epilepsy and art. Med J Aust. 1996;165(1):64.
7. Collins W. Poor Miss Finch. USA: Oxford University Press; 1995.
8. Ladino LD, Hunter G, Téllez-Zenteno JF. Art and epilepsy surgery. Epilepsy Behav. 2013;29(1):82-9.
9. Iris Hauser. [online] Available from http://www.irishauser.ca. [Last accessed January, 2025]
10. Sachter SC. Epilepsy and art: Windows into complexity and comorbidities. Epilepsy Behav. 2016;57(Pt B):265-9.

CHAPTER

7

Migraine and Art

INTRODUCTION

Migraine has a long history. An ancient Babylonian text describes migraine as "Head disease roameth over the desert, blowing like the wind, flashing like lightening, it is loosened above and below, it cutteth off him who feareth not his God like a reech, like a stack of henna it slitteth his threws." "Head disease" made its victim "glow as a star of heaven" so that he would not find peace and "had to run about at night like water." From the description and severity of the pain, it is possible that the description fits in more with cluster headache than migraine. Centuries ago, the Rig Vedas also provided description of migraine like headaches. The exact pathophysiology of migraine is not known fully. However, the role of cortical spreading depression (CSD) has been much highlighted.

Cortical Spreading Depression and Migraine Aura

Cortical spreading depression is thought to be the neurophysiological correlate of migraine and was first described by Aristides Leao in 1944. It is characterized by a slowly (3–5 mm/min) propagating wave of depolarization in neuronal and glial cell membranes that is followed by inhibition of cortical activity for up to 30 minutes, coinciding with the initiation and progression of aura symptoms.[1] The spread normally starts from the occipital region and spreads anteriorly toward the frontal regions.

This wave of spreading depression is also associated with a wave of hyperemia, followed by a prolonged phase of cortical oligemia. CSD is initiated by local elevations in extracellular potassium (K^+) that chronically depolarize neurons for approximately 30–50 seconds. It has been suggested that the initial accumulation of extracellular K^+ occurs as a result of repeated depolarization and repolarization of hyperexcitable neurons in the cerebral cortex, and that this accumulation of extracellular K^+ then further depolarizes the cells from which it was released. This large efflux of K^+ is associated with a major disruption of cell membrane ionic gradients, influx of sodium (Na^+) and calcium (Ca^{++}), and release of glutamate.

The propagation of CSD is still not fully understood, and several hypotheses exist. Originally, the interstitial diffusion of either K^+ or glutamate was thought to lead to the propagation of CSD, but later theories suggest that the propagation is mediated via gap junctions between glial cells or neurons. Increasing evidence from animal studies supports the assumption that CSD can activate trigeminal nociception, and thus trigger headache mechanisms. The question is—does CSD cause the aura symptoms? Probably so. The hypoperfusion of CSD in some way induces both the positive and the negative components of the aura. The next question that arises is whether CSD occurs in subjects with migraine without aura. CSD generation is an integral part of the migraine cascade and probably activates meningeal inflammation and trigeminal nociception through release of noxious chemicals. So, it must occur in subjects with MO as well. It was suggested earlier that CSD in MO principally occurs in silent or noneloquent areas of the cortex and hence no aura symptoms are produced. More recent thoughts are that the CSD in MO does not reach the threshold to produce focal neurological features which we call aura. Two other aspects about CSD propagation need to be considered. CSD spread does not follow vascular territory but stops at major sulci. However, it can bypass major sulcus as well by travelling deep into the depths of the sulcus and then coming back on surface traveling up along the cortex on the other side of the deep sulcus. This can explain the development of both motor and sensory symptoms in subjects with hemiplegic migraine where CSD crosses (passing below) the central sulcus, involving both motor and sensory cortical areas by this mechanism.[1]

The question arises why an essay on migraine art? Leonardo da Vinci wrote in the 15th century *"And you want to demonstrate with words..... do away with such an idea, because the more minutely you describe the more you will confuse the mind of the reader, and the more you will remove him from knowledge of the thing described; it is therefore necessary both to make a drawing of it as well as to describe it"*. Schott published in Brain in 2007[2] an article entitled *"Exploring the visual aura: The tacit contribution of illustration"* which clearly would support Da Vinci's contention. The illustrations depicted in this essay are mostly gathered from the exhibition of Migraine Art held in London, UK from 1980 to 1987 which the author had visited a number of years back.

This essay would discuss the subject under the following heads: Depiction of Migraine Pain in Art; Depiction of Migraine Visual Aura in Art; Depiction of Disorders of Body Image in Migraine in Art; and Art works Inspired by Migraine and Migraine in Literature.

Depiction of Migraine Pain in Art

The following artworks **(Figs. 1A to H)** mostly displayed at the aforementioned exhibition display different types pain location and nature of migraine pain in different artists. The facial appearance of the subjects drawn on the whole would give an idea to the viewers about the intensity of the pain being experienced. One of the drawings showing severe degree of eye pain, as if the eye ball is being pulled out, may be one of cluster headache. Otherwise both holocranial and hemicranial

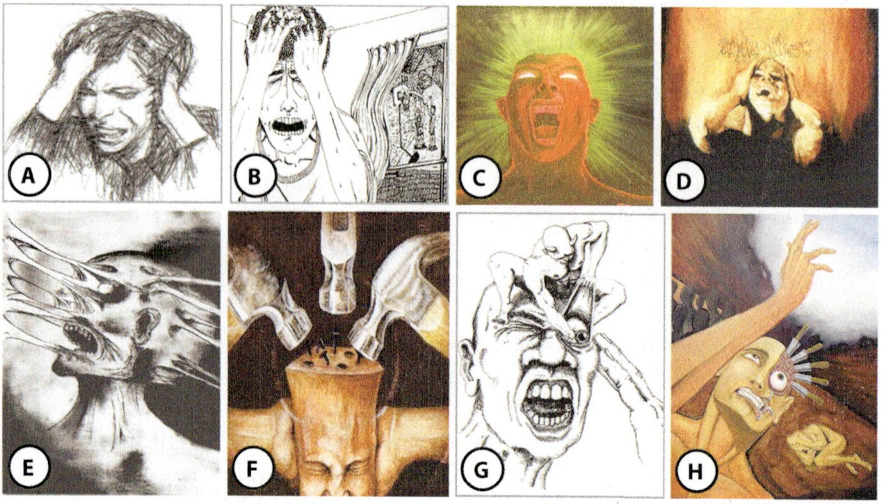

FIGS. 1A TO H: Different types of migraine pain as experienced by patients and their visual artistic expressions of the same.

headaches are being displayed including one subject having pain in the cervical region. Another subject with severe left orbital pain is displayed as lying down in bed in a curled up manner; this is unlikely to be cluster headache where subjects are extremely restless and cannot lie down in bed quietly.

Migraine patients may experience a variety of peculiar pain sensations which are very similar to the spontaneous pain sensations occurring in patients with thalamic lesions and to the cenesthesias described in functional psychotic patients. Podoll et al. in 1999[3] described a 36-year-old artist with a history of migraine with typical aura provided impressive illustrations of cenesthetic pain sensations experienced during his migraine attacks, including sensations of pressure and sensations of pulling. It may be surmised that cenesthetic pain sensations **(Figs. 2A to C)** represent aura symptoms of migraine indicative of focal cerebral dysfunction, possibly in the thalamic region. The occurrence of cenesthetic pain sensations as a migraine symptom supports an organic basis of cenesthesias. The illustrations below depict some such sensations experienced by the artist.

Chakravarty et al. studied migraine pain location in a large sample of both children and adults both at pain onset and then its subsequent spread and location. Significant differences have been noted in migraine pain location between these two groups. Unilateral onset pain is common in adults; side locked and vertex onset pain unusual in children; holocranial onset pain much common in children and cervico-occipital onset pain much less common in children. There have been differences in evolution of migraine pain as well. During established headache, unilateral pain was recorded in only a small proportion of children (10.5%) whereas it was noted in many adults subjects (40.5%).[4]

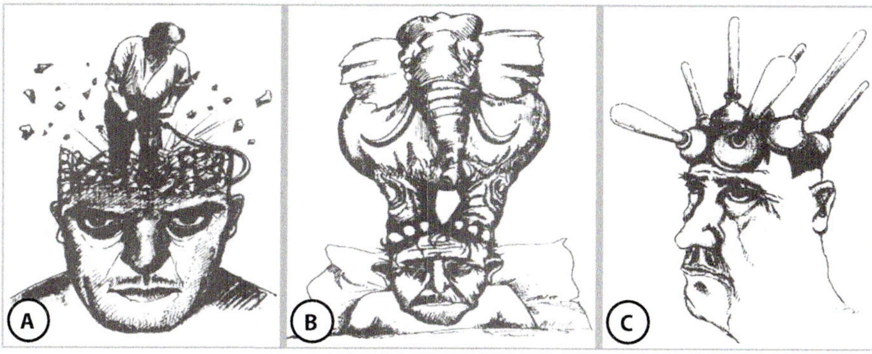

FIGS. 2A TO C: Types of cenesthetic pain sensations.

Depiction of Migraine Visual Aura in Art

The possible pathogenesis of migraine visual aura had been briefly discussed earlier. Classical migraine visual aura takes the form of a zig-zag lines which is often bright and scintillating and generally occurs in one hemifield right or left. This is designated as fortification spectra because of its resemblance to the design of old roman forts in England. The illustrations **(Figs. 3A to C)** below would bring home the point.

Some detailing of the zig-zag lines is provided in the third illustration. *"The bars in the fortification arc show that they consist of two parallel bright lines with a dark gap between. They are shimmering and oscillating in brightness, with all the inside lines 'on' when all outside lines are 'off', and vice versa producing a boiling or rolling motion. This suggested that there is a network of reciprocal inhibition, with depression of activity enhancing the spontaneous neural activity in adjacent regions"* (Richards 1971).[5] Question would remain whether migraine visual auras are illusions or hallucinations?

Joseph Mallord William Turner (23 April 1775 to 19 December 1851), known in his time as *William Turner*, was an English romantic painter, printmaker, and watercolorist. He is known for his expressive coloring, imaginative landscapes, and turbulent, often violent marine paintings. One of Turner's famous water colors is the painting The Piazzetta, Venice **(Fig. 4)**. A crack of lightning streaks the sky above the Piazzetta, the historic heart of government in Venice, and bystanders run for cover. The city of canals captured Turner's imagination more than any other place. Question has been raised whether it was really a lightening or a fortification spectra during one of Turner's migraine aura while he was busy painting the Piazzetta.

Depictions of Distortions Body Image in Migraine Arts[6,7]

Body image (BI) is the model of our body as represented in the brain *(Bonnier)*, different from the anatomical map of the body in the sensory or motor cortex. BI is solely based on different sensations carried to the brain by the sensory systems—

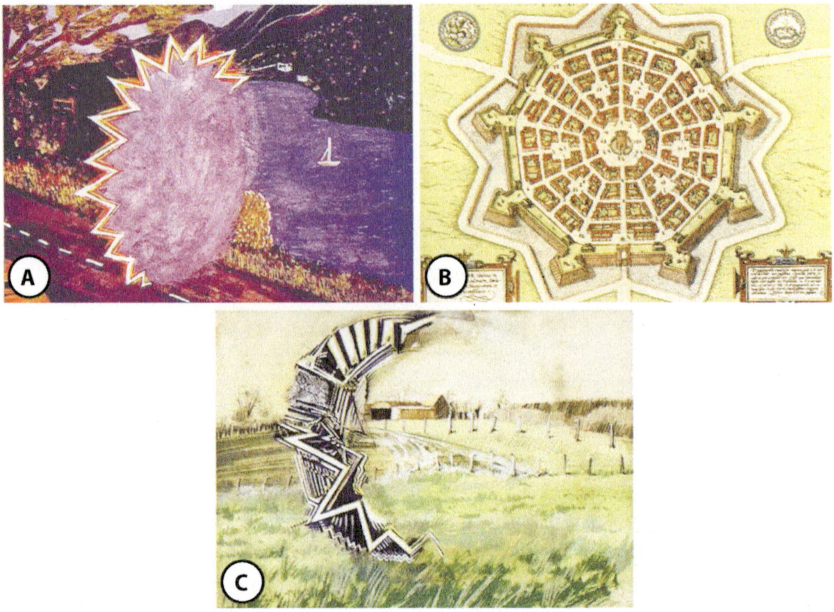

FIGS. 3A TO C: Different types of typical migraine visual auras. Resemblance to Roman Fort.

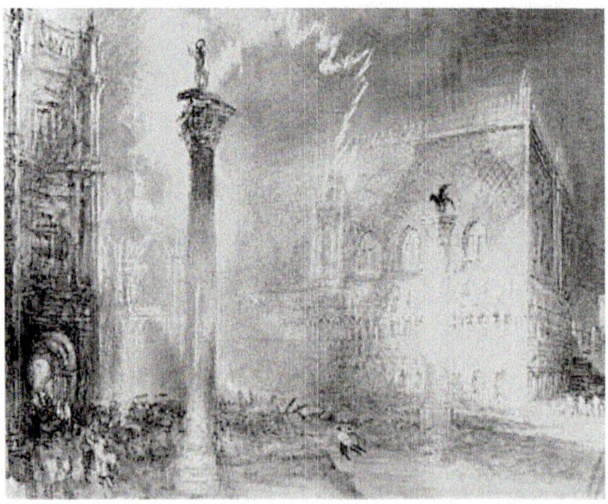

FIG. 4: Turner's painting; The Piazzetta, Venice.

somatic and special. BI is a plastic moldable model varying from time to time as sensations vary and body positions change and limb and body dimensions alter with age. Is it present at birth? BI is a genetically hardwired image hence subjects with phocomelia never complain of phantom limb pain due to absence of the image of the undeveloped body part in the BI. The classical hallucinatory BI disorders are illustrated in **Figure 5**.

The painting below **(Fig. 6)** illustrates the out of body experience of an artist with migraine which developed as a part of an aura along with a classical zig-zag visual aura.

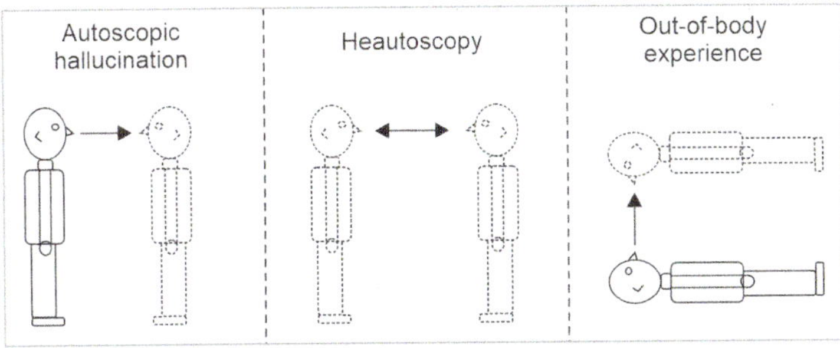

FIG. 5: Symbolic representations of disorders of body image.

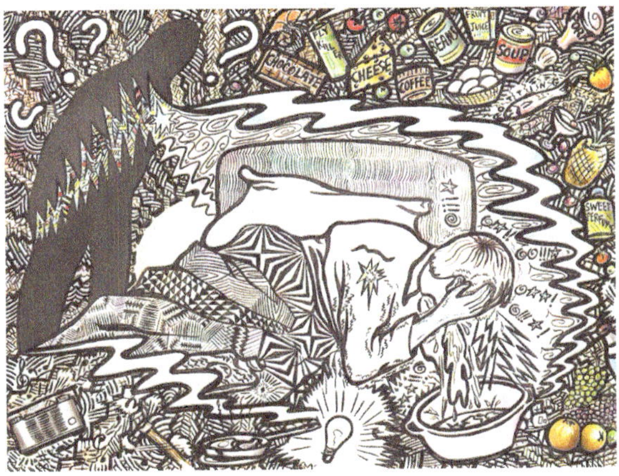

FIG. 6: Out of body experience as migraine aura.

Here, the subject is seen experiencing a bad right hemicranial headache associated with vomiting and he is seen visualizing a zig-zag visual aura in his left visual hemifield. Now watch the black shadowy figure on the left hemifield and looking at the patient. This is a hallucinatory experience of looking at himself from outside his own body—developing as a part of the migraine aura—an out of body experience. Such hallucinatory experience may occur as an epileptic aura and also in survivors who recover from a cardiac arrest. Several types of distortions of one's own body may be visualized during a migraine aura. Some such examples displayed at the London exhibition are shown in **Figures 7A and B**.

Another major form of distortion of BI is splitting of BI resulting in an aura during the face may appear to be split in the middle or much distorted (Mosaic vision) that it may look like a Cubist painting when viewed in a mirror and can later be drawn or painted by expert artists with migraine **(Figs. 8A to D)**.

Because of the similarity of the such split visual auras to some of Pablo Picasso's paintings, question had been raised whether Picasso had suffered from migraine with split vision auras which might have inspired him to innovate the Cubist painting style.[8,9] Opinion remains divided on this issue till date. The term

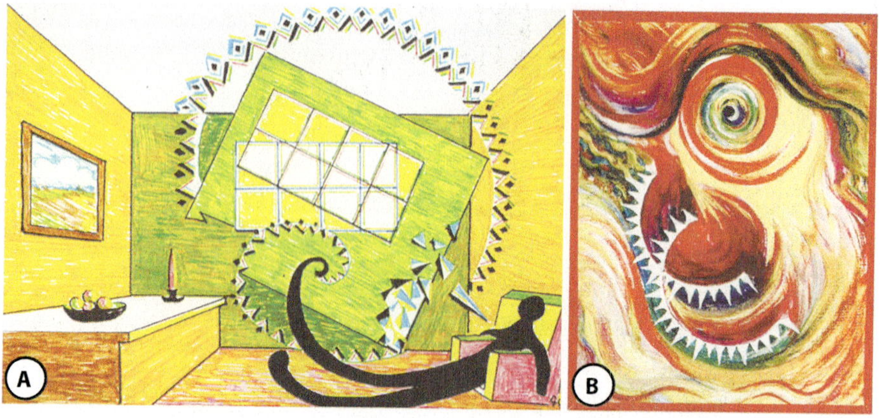

FIGS. 7A AND B: Hallucinatory visual auras.

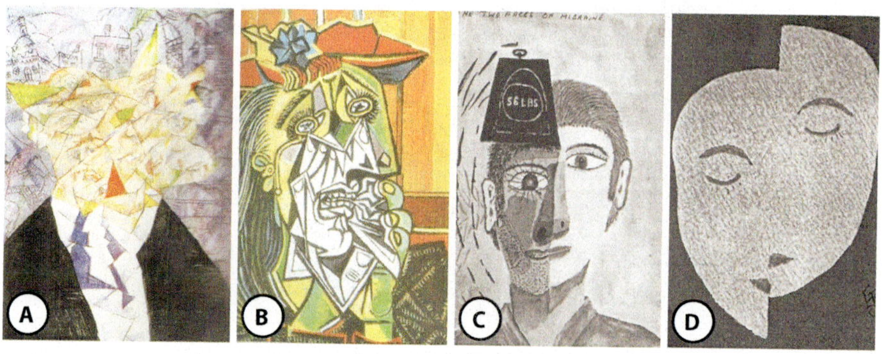

FIGS. 8A TO D: Examples of mosaic vision.

Pablo Picasso syndrome may be applicable to some individuals who notably experience metamorphopsias, or distortions in size (micropsia/macropsia) and distance (teleopsia), particularly of body parts. Some migraineurs, however, report dislocation and disorientation of body parts, which are common features found in paintings of Pablo Picasso.[10] A 60-year-old lady with migraine complained that in-between her attacks of migraine, she would occasionally notice alterations in her visual perceptions which she described as a "Picasso" painting. She would note people's ears on top of their head, or their shortened right arm attached to the face. Such phenomenon would occur 1–2 times per week and would last 5–10 minutes. Nonliving objects would never appear distorted.

Macrosomatognosia and Microsomatognosia in Migraine Art

Robinson and Podoll[11] noted these features in 18 artists with migraine with aura. Macrosomatognosia was more common than microsomatognosia and applied more often to single parts of the body, whereas microsomatognosia mostly affected the whole body. In partial macrosomatognosia, the head and upper extremities are the body parts most frequently involved; their representation in the sensory maps of the human cortex **(Figs. 9 and 10)** is more extensive as well.

Inspired by Migraine Aura

Giorgio de Chirico was a central figure in 20th century art in France. De Chirico suffered from several complaints including spells of abdominal pain, vomiting and headaches. He probably had the periodic syndrome or abdominal migraine. He developed a scotoma associated with fortification spectra. "Other descriptions included sparkling, dazzling, dancing, or flickering lights, fire rings, stars, and dancing lines." He felt these to be spiritual fever and such auras probably had a significant influence on his artworks described as metaphysical.[12] Some examples are given below **(Fig. 11)**.

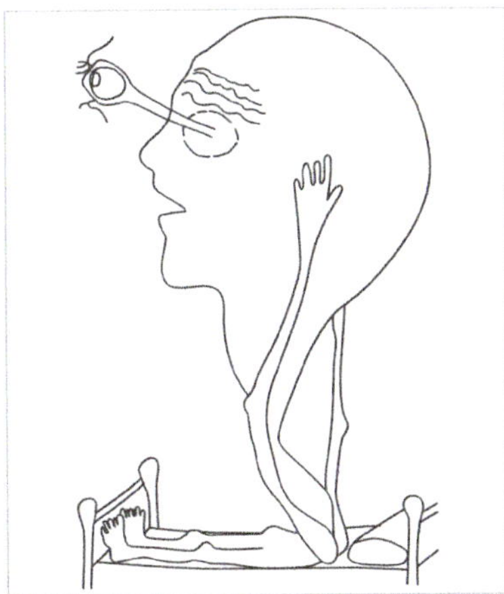

FIG. 9: Macrosomatognosia as migraine visual aura.

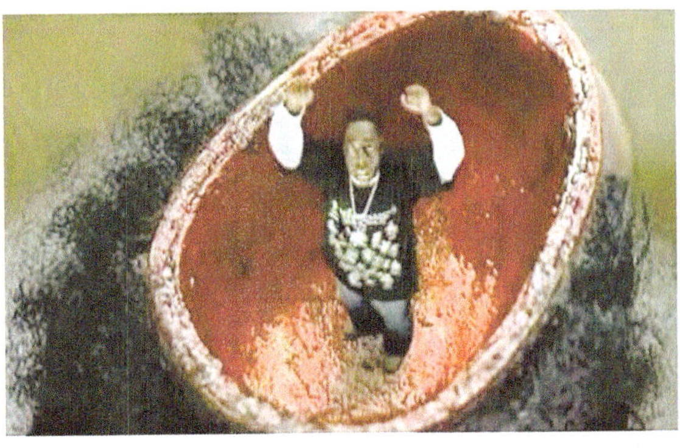

FIG. 10: Microsomatognosia as migraine visual aura.

Blaise Pascal's (1623–1662) Religious Experience (1654)

The writings of Blaise Pascal (1623–1662), a mathematician, physicist (Pascal's law), and theologist, are often thought of as an ideal example of classical French prose. In fact, Pascal had a religious conversion in the 1650s and following this he devoted himself more to religion than science. There is evidence that Pascal suffered from migraine with visual aura with recurring headaches, episodes of blindness in half of his visual field, zig-zag, fortification spectra, and other visual hallucinations. It is believed that the migraine aura experiences might have acted as a source of inspiration for Pascal's philosophical reflections. Pascal's sudden religious conversion, during the night of the 23rd to 24th of November 1654, was accompanied by a lighted vision which he interpreted as fire which brought him the total conviction of God's "reality and presence". This experience may have been based on the effects of a migraine aura attack.[13,14]

Sarah Raphael (1960-2001) was an English painter whose prolonged migraines, lasting as long as 18 months, influenced her work in several ways. Firstly, her paintings incorporate various aspects of her visual auras, including scotomas and objects with photopsias and superimposed zig-zag lines. Secondly, she had increased olfactory sensitivity, to the point that certain components of oil paint triggered attacks. For this reason, she began using odorless acrylic paint. In the artist's own words, she developed a "migraine-friendly" painting style.[15]

Ignatius Brennan (born in 1949) is an Irish painter who is greatly affected with migraine auras. Among his symptoms he describes "geometric figures, zig-zag lines, blurred shapes, tunnel vision or a kaleidoscopic effect, loss of three-dimensional vision, and occasionally a disorder of bodily perception, with a feeling of possessing duplicated limbs". He has creatively incorporated these phenomena into his artworks.[16] Below are some examples **(Figs. 12A to D)**.

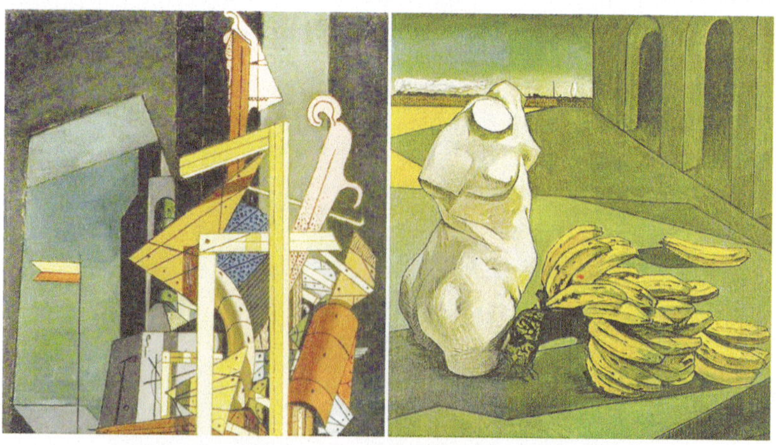

FIG. 11: Metaphysical paintings of Giorgio de Chirico.

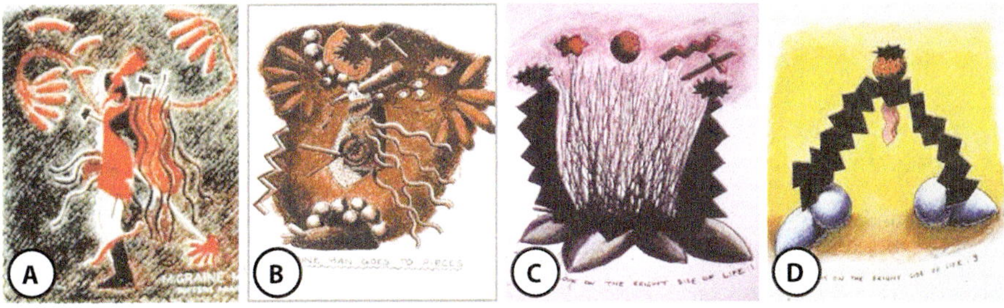

FIGS. 12A TO D: Some paintings of Ignatius Brennan. To note the geometric shapes and kaleidoscopic effect. The zig-zag visual aura impression is retained.

MIGRAINE IN LITERATURE

Alice in Wonderland is an 1865 English children story book by Lewis Carroll, a mathematics professor at Oxford. It describes the experiences of a girl named Alice who fell through a rabbit hole into a fantasy world of strange anthropomorphic creatures. The artist John Tenniel provided 42 wood-engraved illustrations for the book. Lewis Carrol is the pseudonym of Charles Lutwidge Dodgson. There are three stories named: Alice's Adventures in Wonderland, Through the Looking Glass, and What Alice Found There. Two types of hallucinatory experiences are described of probably migraneous in origin. These include—visual hallucination and somesthetic hallucination (BI) with both macropsia and microscopia and distortions.[17,18] Some examples are given below **(Figs. 13A and B)**.

Alice in Wonderland syndrome (AIWS) is a rare condition where there is a conglomeration of symptoms involving altered perception of shape (metamorphosia) of objects or persons who appear to be smaller (micropsia) or larger (macropsia) than normal, of impaired sense of passage of time, and of zooming of the environment. It was first described by Lippmann in 1952 and the literary name was given by Todd in 1955. All of Todd's 6 cases of AIWS had episodic body-image distortions like those experienced by Lewis Carroll's Alice character. Although some also had visual perceptual disturbances, but none had visual perceptual disorders without body-image distortions. Hence, AIWS may be accompanied by visual perceptual disorders (e.g., micropsia, macropsia, teleopsia, and pelopsia), but basing the diagnosis of AIWS on isolated visual perceptual disorders, as has subsequently been done by a number of authors, would not be appropriate. Cases of isolated visual illusions without self-perceived distortions of body size, shape, or form do not meet Todd's original criteria. Furthermore, such cases differ by age and etiology from those that involve somesthetic perceptual disorders. Therefore, the use of the term AIWS for isolated visual illusions is problematic and should be discouraged. Although Todd's and Lippmann's cases were adolescents or adults, AIWS is most commonly reported in children. Reported causes include infection (especially with Epstein-Barr virus), migraine, epilepsy, depression, and toxic and febrile causes of altered mental state.

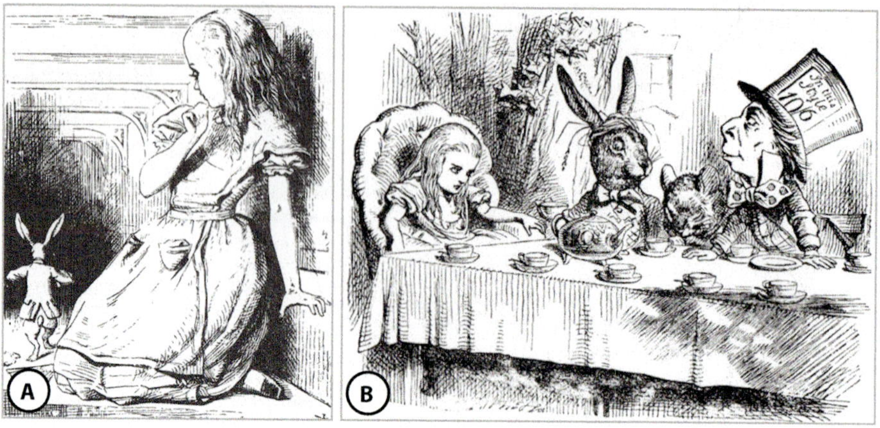

FIGS. 13A AND B: Drawings from Alice in Wonderland.

CONCLUDING REMARKS

This essay portrays the various clinical manifestations of migraine as experienced by artists through their art works. The essay echoes what da Vinci wrote centuries back on the role played by illustrations in learning and teaching. There cannot be a better mode than visual art to narrate the experiences of artist migraineurs experiencing multiple types of auras, visual or otherwise.

REFERENCES

1. Chakravarty A. (2019). Case Studies in Uncommon Headache Disorder. [online] Available from https://books.google.com/books?id=mXKSDwAAQBAJ. [Last accessed January, 2025]
2. Schott GD. Exploring the visual hallucinations of migraine aura: the tacit contribution of illustration. Brain. 2007;130(Pt 6):1690-703.
3. Podoll K, Bollig G, Vogtmann T, Pothmann R, Robinson D. Cenesthetic pain sensations illustrated by an artist suffering from migraine with typical aura. Cephalalgia. 1999;19(6): 598-601.
4. Chakravarty A, Mukherjee A, Roy DJ. Migraine pain location: how do children differ from adults? Headache Pain. 2008;9(6):375-9.
5. Richards W. The Fortification Illusions of Migraines. Sci Am. 1971;224(5):88-96.
6. Podoll K, Robinson D. Out-of-body experiences and related phenomena in migraine art. Cephalalgia. 1999;19(10):886-96.
7. Podoll K, Robinson D. Illusory splitting as visual aura symptom in migraine. Cephalalgia. 2000;20(4):228-32.
8. Haan J, Ferrari MD. Picasso's migraine: Illusory cubist splitting or illusion? Cephalalgia. 2011;31(9):1057-60.
9. Ferrari MD, Haan J. Migraine aura, illusory vertical splitting, and Picasso. Cephalalgia. 2000;20(8):686.
10. Suri R, Ali A. Coining the Pablo Picasso Syndrome. Headache. 2020;60(3):626-9.
11. Robinson D, Podoll K. Macrosomatognosia and microsomatognosia in migraine art. Acta Neurol Scand. 2000;101(6):413-6.

12. Bogousslavsky J. The neurology of art--the example of Giorgio de Chirico. Eur Neurol. 2003;50(4):189-90.
13. Sava A, Dumitrescu M, Dumitrescu GF, Turliuc MD, Ciocoiu M, Scripcariu V. The mysterious "mental illness" of a philosopher: the case of Blaise Pascal. Rom J Morphol Embryol. 2019;60(4):1383-9.
14. Paciaroni M. Blaise Pascal and his visual experiences. Recenti Prog Med. 2011;102(12):494-6.
15. Podoll K, Ayles D. Inspired by migraine: Sarah Raphael's 'Strip!' paintings. J R Soc Med. 2002;95(8):417-9.
16. Piechowski-Jozwiak B, Bogousslavsky J. Neurological diseases in famous painters Prog Brain Res. 2013:203:255-75.
17. Lanska DJ, Lanska JR. The Alice-in-Wonderland Syndrome. Front Neurol Neurosci. 2018;42:142-50.
18. Blom JD. Alice in Wonderland syndrome: A systematic review. Neurol Clin Pract. 2016;6(3):259-70.

CHAPTER

8

The Science of Visual Neglect and Art

INTRODUCTION

Unilateral neglect and inattention are the most striking abnormalities manifested by patients with right hemispheric lesions.[1] Patients with an acute right hemispheric stroke are frequently lying on their right side, with head and eyes turned to the right. They attend to stimuli coming from the right but not the left. A patient may ignore an examiner approaching from the left until he or she crosses into the right visual field. Left hemianopia may or may not be present; some patients can see stimuli in the left visual field but pay no attention to them (visual hemineglect). As noted earlier, a patient with a right hemispheric lesion may neglect the left side of the body when dressing or shaving. They may eat the food on the right side of a plate but leave the left side untouched, stumble onto walls or objects on the left side, leave out words at the beginning of a line while reading, and fail to notice cars coming from the left side. If the subject happens to be an artist, the left half of his paintings or sculptures would be done less meticulously than the right side. Hemineglect, thus, is a deficit of great functional importance in the activities of daily living and it can involve not only body parts but also the surrounding space.

Neglect can be visual, tactile, auditory, and even olfactory related to the contralateral side of the surrounding. A related phenomenon is extinction of the left-sided stimuli when bilateral stimuli are presented—also called perceptual rivalry. Functional MR studies have shown activation of the right occipital cortex in response to left-sided visual stimuli that are extinguished and not consciously seen by the subject; these stimuli are thus perceived cortically but not brought to conscious awareness.

Another striking feature is the rarity of right visual hemineglect related to a left hemispheric lesion. The cause is not clear but may be related to the masking of the neglect by the devastating effects of a left brain stroke with loss of communication.

Anosognosia is a related condition where the neglect of the left side of the body is so deep that some patients may deny having anything wrong with their left limbs. When asked to raise both arms, only the right goes up and the patient may continue to mention that there is no weakness on the left side. Such patients are often totally unconcerned about the paralysis—a condition called anosodiaphoria by Charcot and Babinski. They may, at times, deny that the paralyzed limb actually belongs to them but to someone else and may give a name to that particular limb. Neglects of these kinds are not very uncommon during the acute stage of strokes and significantly interfere with institution of early rehabilitation programs till these show some degree of improvement with time.

When a subject with a presumed stroke ignores one side of his visual field, it is important to differentiate between hemianopia due to a retrochiasmal on the opposite or a visual hemineglect due to lesion on the opposite hemisphere lesion. In general, hemivisual neglect is a transitory phenomenon lasting for few hours to a few days while a hemianopia may be a permanent disability though many patients learn to avoid the field loss by compensatory head movements. The line bisection test is a quick measure to detect the presence of unilateral spatial neglect (visual). To do the test, one must place a mark with a pencil through the center of a series of horizontal lines. Usually, a displacement of the bisection mark toward the side of the brain lesion is interpreted as a symptom of neglect.

Localization of lesions causing left visual hemineglect is complex. Comments had already been made in relation to common occurrence of neglect phenomenon in right hemispheric lesions. Some alteration between the right and left hemispheres may also contribute. The possible sites of lesions in the right hemisphere causing left visual hemineglect are shown in **Figure 1**. Lesions in the inferior parietal lobule consisting of the angular and supramarginal gyri commonly cause left visual hemineglect, at least temporarily. The temporoparietal junction is very critical. Additionally, lesions as far forward as the medial and inferior frontal gyri may also be relevant. If neglect occurs in left hemispheric aphasic patients, it generally occurs due to pressure effect on the right hemispheric structures or through interruption of ascending and descending pathways in the brainstem again due to shift and coning.

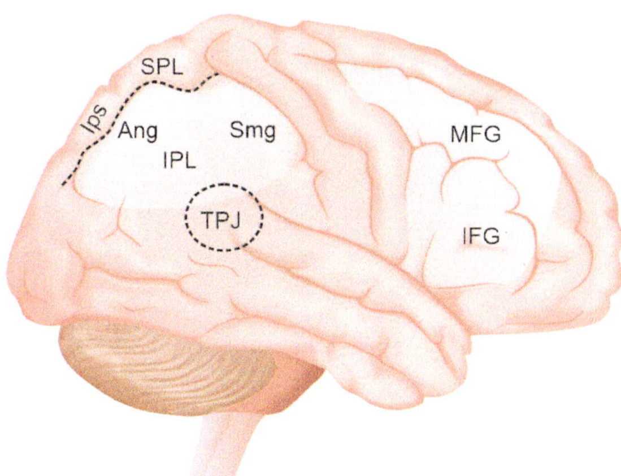

FIG. 1: Brain areas lesions of which can produce visual hemineglect on the opposite side.
(TPJ: temporoparietal junction; IFG: inferior frontal gyrus; MFG: middle frontal gyrus; IPL: inferior frontal lobule; Ang: angular gyrus; Smg: supramarginal gyrus; SPL: superior parietal lobule)

Artists with right hemispheric strokes

- Loss of contours
- Misplacement of details
- Neglect and obscuring of texture
- Loss of emotional closeness
- Increased subjectivity
- Obscurity and blurriness
- Dissimilarity of familiar faces in portraits
- Asymmetry and distortion of faces in portraits and self-portraits
- Lack of correct perspective
- Anatomical curiosities and lack of anatomical exactitude

EFFECTS OF HEMINEGLECT ON ARTWORKS

Strokes are the most common cause of development of visual neglect seen in clinical practice. Focal lesions such as strokes significantly affect painting production in the vast majority of artists. In particular, painters, when they resume painting, show changes in their painting style. In exceptional cases, there may be an apparent improvement in style, but in most cases, the changes represent nothing short of deterioration. Several observations have been made on artists who suffered from right brain strokes. These include[2]

The pre- and post-stroke paintings of four famous European artists depict many of the aforementioned features including left visual hemineglect especially in cases of Lovis Corinth and Federico Fellini who was also a famous actor **(Figs. 2 to 5)**. The first painting made by Lovis Corinth after recovery from a right posterior parietal infarct clearly shows a left visual hemineglect as right half of the lady is much poorly done compared to the other side.

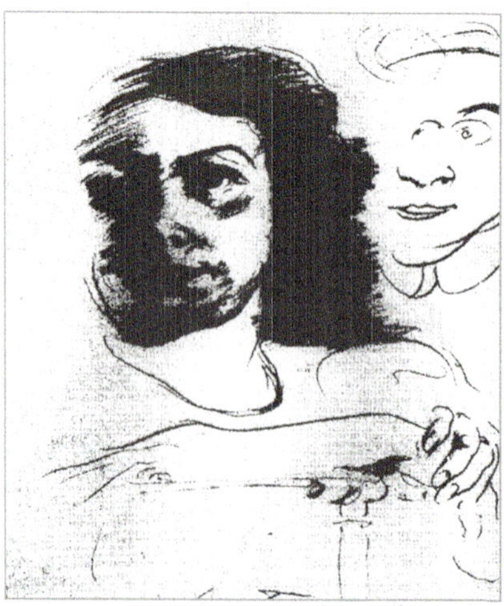

FIG. 2: Lovis Corinth (1858–1927): Painting of his wife.

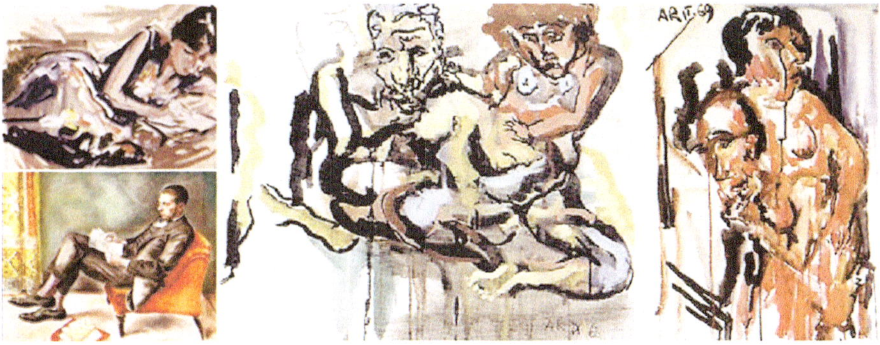

FIG. 3: Anton Räderscheidt (1892–1970): Pre- and post-stroke (1967) paintings.

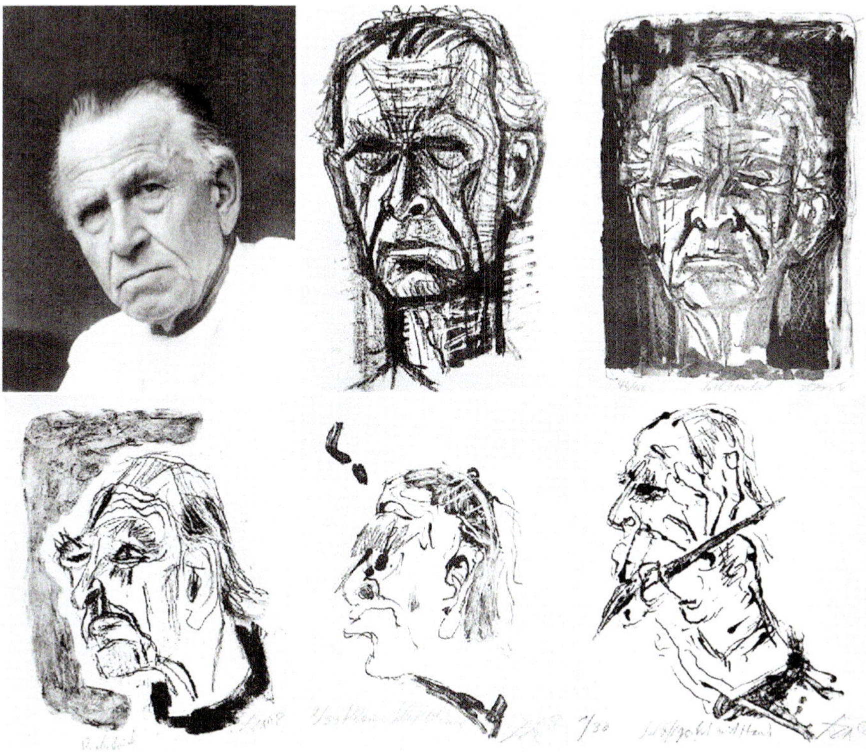

FIG. 4: Otto Dix (1891–1969): Pre- and post-stroke (1967) self-portraits.

Personal Experience

A 46-year-old IIT Professor of Design (right handed), also an accomplished painter, had a right parietal ischemic stroke in 2009. He recovered reasonably well over next several months. He had residual left arm weakness with spasticity but started working and was made HOD. He was attending international meetings and

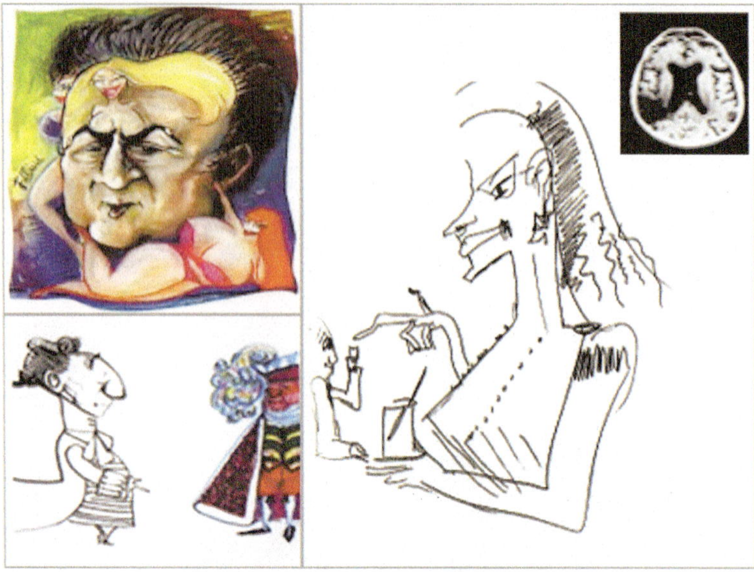

FIG. 5: Federico Fellini (1920–1993): Pre- and post-stroke (1993) paintings.

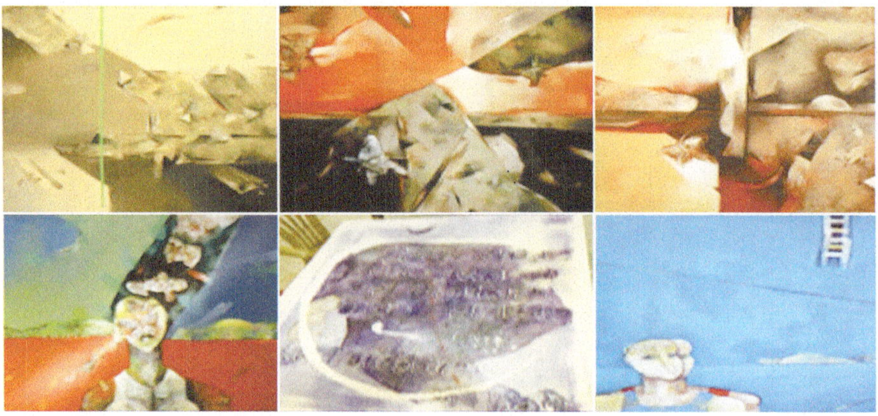

FIG. 6: Pre- and post-stroke paintings of the aforementioned patient.

workshops, and started painting (age 53). His pre-stroke paintings were mostly abstract ones of high quality. Post-stroke, the paintings were more figurative, realistic and, childish and were of much lower quality aesthetically **(Fig. 6)**.

Visual hemineglect may develop following subarachnoid hemorrhage (described by Lythgoe et al.)[3] in a patient who harbored bilateral middle cerebral aneurysms. In the diagram below, the right breast of the girl is missing and right side of the painted face is distorted **(Fig. 7)**.

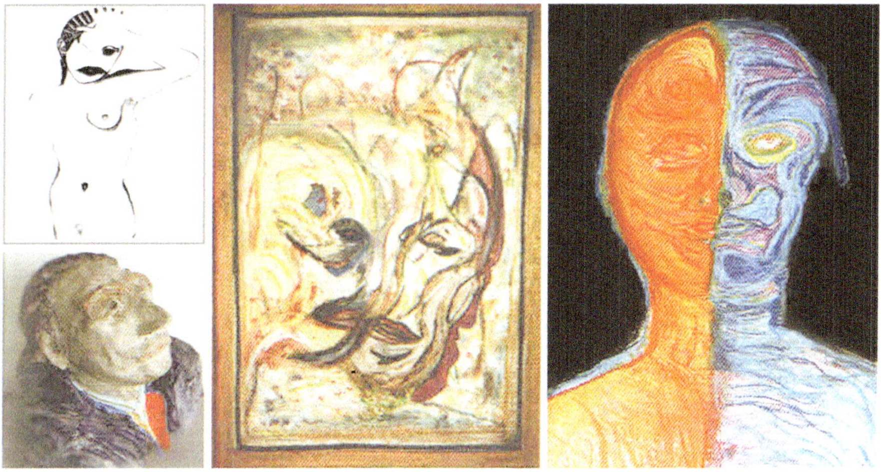

FIG. 7: Left visual hemineglect following subarachnoid hemorrhage.

EVIDENCE OF VISUAL HEMINEGLECT IN AN ARCHAEOLOGICAL SPECIMEN?[4]

In March 2009, the Directorate of Archaeology and Museums of the Government of West Bengal, India, conducted archaeological excavations in the northern Bengal district of Murshidabad and excavated several metal and terracotta objects dating back to the time of the Pala dynasty which ruled Bengal around the 6th century. Of the various objects excavated, was a stucco (a mixture of sand, brick dust, and stone dust) head detached from its body (a statuette). The excavation findings were reported in a national daily (The Telegraph, March 20, 2009). By kind courtesy of the Directorate of Archaeology and Museums, the author had an opportunity to examine this detached stucco head **(Fig. 8)** in detail.

The head was brick red in color and measured about 6 cm in length. Close examination revealed that the left half of the specimen (viewer's left) was beautifully curved, especially the left eye and carvings on the head (possibly curly hair) and it appeared that the stucco head had belonged to a sculpture of a female. The lower portion of the right half of the face (viewer's right) was broken. But although the upper portion remained intact, it showed rather poor artistic carvings. The eye was ill formed and the carvings on the head (so well done on the left side) were virtually absent. The back of the head was broken.

The author argues that the ill-curved right portion of this stucco head most likely represents the work of an artisan who suffered from right visuospatial hemineglect. It is surmised that this resulted from a fairly localized lesion in the left parietotemporal region (cortex or deep white matter) of the artisan which spared the motor cortex as the motor skill of the artisan is quite obvious noting the exquisite carvings on the left portion of the specimen. It is argued that the artisan probably had an ischemic pathology from occlusion of the posterior branch of the left middle cerebral artery. It is highly unlikely that the specimen was the work

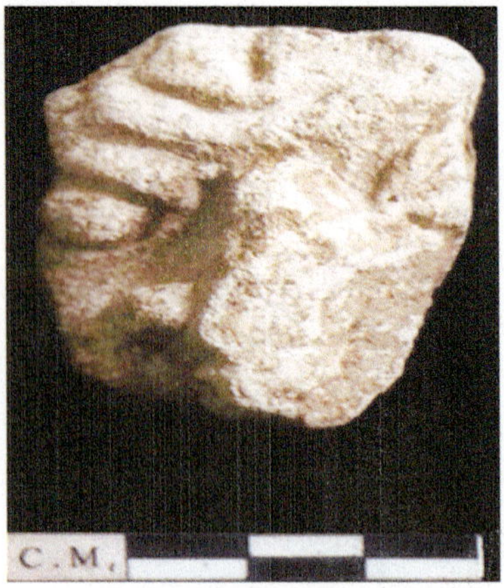

FIG. 8: The sculptures head showing poorly made left side suggestive of a right visual hemineglect in the artisan.

of an artisan with right hemianopia as in that case the right half would not have been sculptured at all. Furthermore, although it might be possible that the age of the specimen and the very process of excavation played a role, the sculpturing difference between the left half and the intact portion of the right half (viewer's) was quite striking for the author to hypothesize on the phenomenon of right hemineglect in the artisan being portrayed in the stucco head specimen.

Mistakes made by the ancient artisans are evident in some archaeological artifacts. Notable example is the major rock edict of Ashoka the Great (304 BC–232 BC) at Jonnagiri in Kurnool district, India. In this, one of the edicts out of 14 was inscribed on the rock on a hillock. The artisan inscribed the words from right to left as is the practice in the case of Kharosthi inscriptions of Ashoka. But Jonnagiri was in Brahmi script and should have been inscribed from left to right and the mistake was attributed to the fact that the artisan was illiterate and probably was used to writing Kharosthi inscriptions on stones.

In the present report, however, the ill-sculptured right half of the stucco head most likely resulted from a neurological deficit in the artisan. Right visuospatial hemineglect is uncommon but can certainly occur. If the hypothesis proposed here is correct, the present specimen (the stucco head) may be considered as the earliest example of the phenomenon of visuospatial hemineglect in an artist.

RIGHT VISUAL HEMINEGLECT IN AN ARTIST WITH BRAIN TUMOR?

A 72-year-old right-handed artist developed a rapidly growing tumor in the left posterior parietal lobe which resulted in bilateral neglect and constructional apraxia that were greater on the right side of his painting than on the left.[5] These changes indicate that a left posterior parietal lesion alters visuospatial perception and constructional ability on both sides of a painting with the contralateral hemispace more impaired than the ipsilateral **(Fig. 9)**.

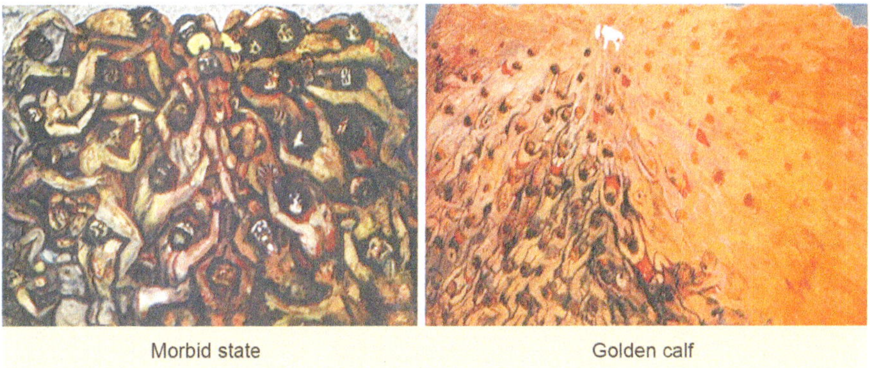

FIG. 9: Right visual hemineglect in a patient with left parietal glioma.

CONCLUDING REMARKS

Unilateral spatial (hemi-)neglect or (hemi-)inattention are clinical terms used to describe a number of different clinical symptoms which have in common the patient's failure to attend to, respond adequately to, or orient voluntarily to people or objects in the contralateral space. Unilateral spatial neglect is most often observed following brain lesions affecting the right hemisphere, and in particular the right inferior parietal cortex (angular and supramarginal gyrus) and right temporoparietal junction. Generally, the patient's deficit is supramodal: patients with hemineglect fail to respond to novel or meaningful stimuli irrespective of whether they are presented in the visual, auditory, and somesthetic (somatosensory) domain. Several established artists displayed evidence of visual hemineglect when they were afflicted with unilateral, usually right, brain lesions, mostly strokes.

REFERENCES

1. Krishner HS. Disorders of the right hemisphere. Behavioral Neurology: Practical Science of Mind and Brain. Boston: Butterworth-Heinemann; 2012. pp. 159-78.
2. Bazner H, Hennerici MG. Painting after right hemisphere stroke case studies of professional artists. In: Bogousslavsky J, Hennerici MG (Eds). Neurological Disorders of Famous Artists. Basel: Karger; 2007. pp. 1-13.
3. Lythgoe MF, Pollak TA, Kalmus M, De Haan M, Chong WK. Obsessive, prolific artistic following subarachnoid hemorrhage. Neurology. 2005;64:397-8.
4. Chakravarty A. Evidence of visual hemineglect in an archeological specimen? Neurol India. 2009;57(5):674-6.
5. Marsh GG, Philwin B. Unilateral Neglect and Constructional Apraxia in a Right-Handed Artist with A Left Posterior Lesion. Cortex. 1987;23(1):149-55.

CHAPTER

9

Art and Creativity in Parkinson's Disease

INTRODUCTION

Parkinson's disease (PD) is a neurodegenerative disease principally of the central nervous system (CNS) associated with progressive loss of dopaminergic neurons in the pars compacta of the substantia nigra and, thus, reducing the brain's ability to produce and utilize dopamine in the basal ganglionic circuits. Clinically manifesting a wide range of symptoms, the pathological hallmark is the accumulation of Lewy bodies—abnormal aggregates of α-synuclein protein—which develop inside nerve cells in cortical and subcortical structures. PD is generally first clinically diagnosed by the presence of cardinal motor features including bradykinesia (slowness), tremor, and rigidity (stiffness), and associated with damage to the ventral substantia nigra pars compacta (vSNc). Neuronal loss in the ventral substantia nigra also leads to dysfunction in both the mesolimbic and mesocortical pathways. The mesolimbic pathway is connected to the ventral striatum (notably nucleus accumbens, NAcc), associated with motivation and reward seeking/learning, hippocampus (memory formation, navigation, and emotion regulation), ventromedial prefrontal, and orbitofrontal cortices (motivation, reward response, and reward processing). The mesocortical pathway reaches prefrontal cortices, especially dorsolateral regions, related to executive functions, emotional/reward response regulation or judgment. Nonmotor features may begin earlier to motor symptoms in some patients. PDs, much like with frontotemporal dementia (FTD)/frontotemporal lobar degeneration (FTLD), have been described to be associated with spontaneous increases in creativity, as well as in new artistic interest or desire to make art. Some such changes may potentially be related to interaction between both neurodegeneration and treatment via levodopa and, especially, dopamine agonist therapy. Such phenomena may especially be seen in cases where individuals have relatively minor motor problems and/or some specific pattern of dysfunction in mesolimbic pathway regions, and where dopamine agonist usage (targeting specifically D2/D3 receptors) leads to overactivation in these areas, leading to artistic or creative change as well as potential stylistic manifestations such as obsession or punding.

Elsewhere, the present author defined "creativity" as the ability to generate ideas that are both novel and useful or influential in a particular social setting.[1] "Artistic creativity" can be defined as the ability to produce innovative aesthetic works. The link between neuropsychiatric illness and creativity, specially artistic creativity,[2-4] the emergence of talent after temporal damage,[5] stroke,[6] or FTD have long been discussed.[5,7,8] However, enhanced artistic creativity or creative drive has only recently been attributed to PD, a disease posing a paradox for *augmented* creative behavior, since PD is classically characterized by the *reduction* in the motor and executive capabilities.

ENHANCEMENT OF ARTISTIC CREATIVITY IN PARKINSON'S DISEASE: EVIDENCE FROM CASE STUDIES

Contrary to the initial belief of a possible loss in artistic skills[9] in artists who developed Parkinsonian features later in life, a Parkinson Art Project, evaluating the work of 40 artists, demonstrated no decline in visual artistic capacity in artists who become parkinsonian. In fact, several patients with enhanced visual artistic capabilities were reported while under dopaminergic treatment.

The Form of Art

Although the style or category of art, music or literature was not specifically and systematically studied in PD patients, there were pictures, sculptures, novels, and poetry reported demonstrating high-quality work. Schrag et al.[10] described a PD patient who never wrote before, but belonged to a family of poets, who then composed poems that won in an annual contest of the International Association of Poets after being on dopamine agonist agent. Bindler et al.[11] described a patient who had no previous writing talent, developed literary writing skills; he published a historical book that won a literary prize. These workers also described another patient who was beautifully embroidering napkins and also developed writing skills worthy of being broadcasted in the radio.

In the field of visual arts, Walker et al.[12] observed a patient with prior painting skills who produced excessive amounts of pastels under dopamine agonists which was well appreciated in his town due to it being naïve, voluminous, and having a strong sense of color. Chatterjee et al.[13] treated a 68-year-old graphic designer who felt an urge for painting under dopaminergic treatment. His drawing often used vivid colors. Surprisingly, the patient reported motor improvement while drawing, feeling "in complete control, despite being frustratingly impaired in other contexts" (bradykinetic, rigid, tremor, and micrographia). During painting, his hand movements were free and controlled with no freezing even while making large amplitude winding movements. The specific artistic style he adopted emphasized larger amplitude proximal movements that were relatively preserved while graphic impairment was evident with distal movements. Why does this discrepancy occur between spontaneous movements (bradykinesia) and movements happening during painting? Chatterjee et al.[13] hypothesized that a possible reason for this discrepancy might be related to differences in proximal versus distal target reaching during painting. This might be similar to the phenomenon of kinesia paradoxa observed in some patients with PD.

Pinker[14] mentioned the paintings of Dr Johanne Vermette, an artist and physician with PD, who wrote "The new style is less precise but more vibrant....I have a need to express myself more". Pinker[14] felt that medication may play a role in enhancing imagination and thus enhance creative output.

The Effect of Predominantly Affected Body Side

Canesi et al.[15] studied 18 PD patients with enhanced creativity and found no correlation between side of disease onset and creativity indices using the Torrance test of creative thinking. Drago et al.,[16] however, found a decrease in verbal creativity not related to decreased fluency.

Schrag et al.,[10] as mentioned earlier, described a patient with novel poetic skills while on dopamine agonist therapy argued whether a possible implicating mechanism could be hypergraphia; however, hypergraphia per se would have no meaningful content which was not the case of this patient.

Effects of Deep Brain Stimulation

Drago et al.[16,17] described a lady who after left subthalamic nucleus–deep brain stimulation (STN-DBS) complained that being on DBS interfered with her artistic creativity and art appreciation in way of her art works being more realistic, less colorful, and less abstract. Furthermore, while "on" left DBS, versus "off" DBS, there were significant reductions in her appreciation of artistic technique. When DBS was switched "on", her creativity index was below average.

Another patient who underwent DBS which was placed on the dorsal border zone of the STN developed an urge for nude paintings while his prior taste for painting included architectural figures only.[18]

IS AUGMENTED CREATIVITY IN PARKINSON'S DISEASE MEDICATION/DOSE RELATED OR IS IT PART OF DOPAMINE DYSREGULATION SYNDROME?

Dopamine dysregulation syndrome (DDS) is part of impulse control disorders (ICDs), a serious and well-recognized complication of dopamine replacement therapy which comprises compulsive gambling, buying, sexual behavior, hobbyism, hoarding (the acquisition and failure to discard a large number of items of little or no objective value), and punding—repetitive, purposeless behaviors characterized by an intense preoccupation with specific items or activities like arranging or dismantling objects. Bindler et al.[11] described a patient who wrote a prize-winning book on historical research while his daily medications (including a dopamine agonist) were augmented up to a fairly high level. He developed features of DDS and underwent DBS and lowering of the dose of dopaminergic drugs and this led to the loss of his "writing talent". A second patient examined by the Bindler et al. also showed a dependency between writing talents and treatment namely the dosage of dopaminergic drugs.

Kulisevsky et al.[19] described an amateur artist with PD who had lessened interest in art a few months prior to PD diagnosis and developed better skills after the initiation of therapy at a moderately lower dosage of levodopa. This, however, increased very significantly after addition of a dopamine agonist, cabergoline. He showed no DDS symptoms or other impulsive behavior. On stopping cabergoline, there was a pause in painting. Increase in dosage of levodopa alone was not effective in returning him to paint. It was the initiation of the dopamine agonist pramipexole that the patient resumed painting, and even progressed to a level where he could sell his art for earning. If creativity in PD is part of DDS, this would imply that creative patients show a tendency for impaired impulse control. PD patients who showed enhancement of artistic work after starting dopaminergic treatment and spent most of the time pursuing their newly acquired artistic talents, disregarding their social life and daily duties, may actually resemble subjects with compulsive behavior and punding.[20] However, creative drive, which arose in some PD patients after the introduction of dopaminergic therapy, was not associated with enhanced impulsivity or impulse control deficit suggesting that dopaminergic treatment is unlikely to be considered a definitive cause for the occurrence of any pathological repetitive behavior.[15] However, some may exhibit a peculiar change in the painting content. The post-DBS patient, discussed earlier, was an architect who frequently painted on architectural themes before surgery, with no other painting styles. While he became more creative, he developed an urge for painting nude figures under levodopa and cabergoline treatment which lessened with drug dosage reduction. In a playwright with PD, dopaminergic therapy enhanced his capacities in writing at the cost of him developing ICD symptoms. These lessened after introduction of levodopa with clozapine. There does not seem to be any difference in the frequency of development of DDS features between ergot and non-ergot derived dopamine agonists.

PROPOSED MECHANISMS OF CREATIVITY IN PARKINSON'S DISEASE

A possible mechanism is disinhibition in a way reminiscent of the artistic skills emerging in FTD.[5,8]

Can this disinhibition is behavioral and creativity is a part of impulsivity? Not all patients with enhanced artistic creativity demonstrated symptoms of ICD as mentioned earlier. It was proposed that, in addition to intelligence, domain-specific knowledge and special skills, necessary prerequisites for creativity—divergent thinking, novelty seeking behavior, some degree of suppression of latent inhibition, and a subtle degree of frontal dysfunction are also required.[1] In PD, however, some of newly emergent artists had no prior artistic skills[10] or high intelligence.[10] Novelty seeking behavior can be a positive trait leading to creativity.[1,21] Bodi et al.[22] found that young, never-medicated PDs exhibit markedly reduced novelty seeking and reward processing. Dopamine agonists such as pramipexole and ropinirole increased both novelty seeking and reward processing. Reduced latent inhibition, which is the capacity of the brain to filter irrelevant stimuli from conscious awareness, is supposed to be the biological basis of creativity that facilitates original recombinant ideation. High dopamine levels may disrupt latent inhibition[1] via alterations in the mesolimbic and mesocortical dopaminergic pathways, which are involved in the modulation.

CONCLUDING REMARKS

Artistic talent may emerge in art-naïve PD patients treated by levodopa and dopamine agonists as part of DDS or without such accompanying symptoms. Such skills, in moderation, may improve the quality of life of PD patients. Systematic studies with consecutive patient interviews using validated creativity scales are mandatory to detect the risk factors and extent of this phenomenon in PD and restless legs syndrome treated with dopamine agonists. Functional MRI studies during creative artistic ideation or during any form of creative work may be helpful for the visualization of involved networks in PD patients. The understanding of the special constellation that enables this creative emergence in PD patients may shed light on the brain mechanism of creativity.

REFERENCES

1. Chakravarty A. The creative brain--revisiting concepts. Med Hypotheses. 2010;74(3):606-12.
2. Andreasen NC. Creativity and mental illness: prevalence rates in writers and their first-degree relatives. Am J Psychiatry. 1987;144(10):1288-92.
3. Blumer D. The illness of Vincent van Gogh. Am J Psychiatry. 2002;159(4):519-26.
4. Kyaga S, Lichtenstein P, Boman M, Hultman C, Langstrom N, Landen M. Creativity and mental disorder: family study of 300,000 people with severe mental disorder. Br J Psychiatry. 2011;199(5):373-9.
5. Miller BL, Ponton M, Benson DF, Cummings JL, Mena I. Enhanced artistic creativity with temporal lobe degeneration. Lancet. 1996;348(9043):1744-5.
6. Bogousslavsky J. Artistic creativity, style and brain disorders. Eur Neurol. 2005;54(2):103-11.
7. Mell JC, Howard SM, Miller BL. Art and the brain: the influence of frontotemporal dementia on an accomplished artist. Neurology. 2003;60(10):1707-10.
8. Miller BL, Cummings J, Mishkin F, Boone K, Prince F, Ponton M, et al. Emergence of artistic talent in frontotemporal dementia. Neurology. 1998;51(4):978-82.
9. Lakke JP. Art and Parkinson's disease. Adv Neurol. 1999;80:471-9.
10. Schrag A, Trimble M. Poetic talent unmasked by treatment of Parkinson's disease. Mov Disord. 2001;16(6):1175-6.
11. Bindler L, Anheim M, Tranchant C, Vidailhet P. La créativité du patient parkinsonien. Ann Médico-psychol, Revue Psychiatr. 2011;169(2):104-7.
12. Walker RH, Warwick R, Cercy SP. Augmentation of artistic productivity in Parkinson's disease. Mov Disord. 2006;21(2):285-6.
13. Chatterjee A, Hamilton RH, Amorapanth PX. Art produced by a patient with Parkinson's disease. Behav Neurol. 2006;17(2):105-8.
14. Pinker S. Art movements. Can Med Assoc J. 2002;166(2):224.
15. Canesi M, Rusconi ML, Isaias IU, Pezzoli G. Artistic productivity and creative thinking in Parkinson's disease. Eur J Neurol. 2012;19(3):468-72.
16. Drago V, Foster PS, Okun MS, Haq I, Sudhyadhom A, Skidmore FM, et al. Artistic creativity and DBS: a case report. J Neurol Sci. 2009;276(1-2):138-42.
17. Drago V, Foster PS, Skidmore FM, Heilman KM. Creativity in Parkinson's disease as a function of right versus left hemibody onset. J Neurol Sci. 2009;276(1-2):179-83.

18. Witt K, Krack P, Deuschl G. Change in artistic expression related to subthalamic stimulation. J Neurol. 2006;253(7):955-6.
19. Kulisevsky J, Pagonabarraga J, Martinez-Corral M. Changes in artistic style and behaviour in Parkinson's disease: dopamine and creativity. J Neurol. 2009;256(5):816-9.
20. Fasano A, Petrovic I. Insights into pathophysiology of punding reveal possible treatment strategies. Mol Psychiatry. 2010;15(6):560-73.
21. Djamshidian A, O'Sullivan SS, Wittmann BC, Lees AJ, Averbeck BB. Novelty seeking behaviour in Parkinson's disease. Neuropsychologia. 2011;49(9):2483-8.
22. Bodi N, Keri S, Nagy H, Moustafa A, Myers CE, Daw N, et al. Reward-learning and the novelty-seeking personality: a between- and within-subjects study of the effects of dopamine agonists on young Parkinson's patients. Brain. 2009;132(Pt 9):2385-95.

CHAPTER 10

Dementia and Art

INTRODUCTION

Of all human achievements, visual art would stand among the highest as it provides a means of emotional, aesthetic, and cultural communication with people around. Starting from the upper Paleolithic period where it may have been linked to the emergence of fully human cognition, the trend is continuing till date. Therefore, its neural mechanisms are of scientific interest, and important insights have been provided by clinical studies of artists developing brain disease. Studies done initially focused on discreet neurological lesions, e.g., examining the relative contribution of lesions like strokes in the left or right hemisphere, and deficits of specific functions such as visuospatial attention and the artistic consequence of right- or left-sided visual hemineglect. While focusing on discreet lesions in localized brain regions, such studies failed to capture deficits of higher functions and faculties that are much more diffuse and generalized in nature as in the cases of dementias. Number of case reports published in later years of artists and nonartists with different dementias and reviews have enriched our knowledge about clinically relevant perceptual and cognitive changes in such individuals.

Some attention has also been given to the possibility that a specific perceptual or cognitive deficit in an artist might either enhance or diminish a given aspect of their artwork.

The range of hypothesized functions underlying art production relevant to dementia may be broadly divided into two broad categories:[1]

1. *Those primarily related to the execution of the artwork itself*: Tremor and rigidity in dementias with associated parkinsonian symptoms [e.g., dementia with Lewy bodies (DLB)], apraxia in those with pronounced parietal or frontal involvement [e.g., Alzheimer's disease (AD)], and motor weakness following stroke (e.g., VaD); color perception defects in AD as also the appreciation of the emotional aspects of the subject/object to be painted (a face for example) and lastly memory deficits—recent, past, semantic, and executive/motor planning.

2. *Those related to the creative process*: Creative idea based on representation/memory/knowledge; emotional themes from unexpected sources; planned emotional impact cognitive themes developed with understanding of artistic and cultural context. Needs involvement of limbic, orbitofrontal and insular cortex as well as for cognitive need involvement of prefrontal cortex for executive functions and occipital, temporal, and parietal cortex for stored knowledge.

Deliberate exploration of the cognitive brain is more relevant to scientific creativity; however, it applies to art where an artist actively seeks new ways of representation or chooses to change style or sets out to provoke emotion. Opening a window to the artworks of patients with different types of dementias would bring forth a concept how the aforementioned processes would be modified in diseased states.

ART IN ALZHEIMER'S DISEASE INCLUDING DEVELOPMENT OF DE NOVO ARTISTRY

The condition in which *de novo* artistic behaviors are encountered more commonly is frontotemporal dementia (FTD), mostly of the semantic type.[2] In contrast, in the more common form of dementia namely AD, deterioration in drawing abilities had been well documented.[3] Case reports of artists with AD reveal a declining ability to represent subject matter in a representative fashion.[4] Some of the painter Willem de Kooning's (1904–1997) most celebrated works were made after the onset of AD. Paintings made during the advanced stages of his AD were, however, only composed of formless sheets of color and lines.[5] Cummings and Zarit followed the course of an artist with AD over a 30 months period.[6] His paintings became more simplified and primitive; color palette became progressively restricted and shading and perspectives were lost. Crutch and co-workers[7] studied progressive decline in artistic ability in William Utermohlen, an artist who mostly painted portraits and developed probable AD. There was difficulty in accurately representing individual facial features, both in terms of their structures and spatial relations as also alteration in sense of proportion. Later on, portraits became more abstract looking.

The author reports here the case of a patient with probable AD, who showed de novo development of artistic talents 4 years after the onset of AD-suggestive symptoms and having no previous interest or training in arts.

An 82-year-old right-handed female was first met by the author, in an art exhibition held in connection with the Annual Meeting of the Alzheimer's Disease Society of India in December, 2009. Seven of her paintings were displayed of which two are reproduced here **(Figs. 1 and 2)**. She had no interest or training in art in the past and all these paintings (and many more) were made over the past 4 years. About 8 years back, this lady started having progressive memory loss for mostly recent events which was soon followed by getting lost inside her house and on the road, disorientation in time and place, and difficulty in naming and recognizing her relatives. Her communication skills were retained. About 3 years after the onset of her symptoms, medical consultations were made and

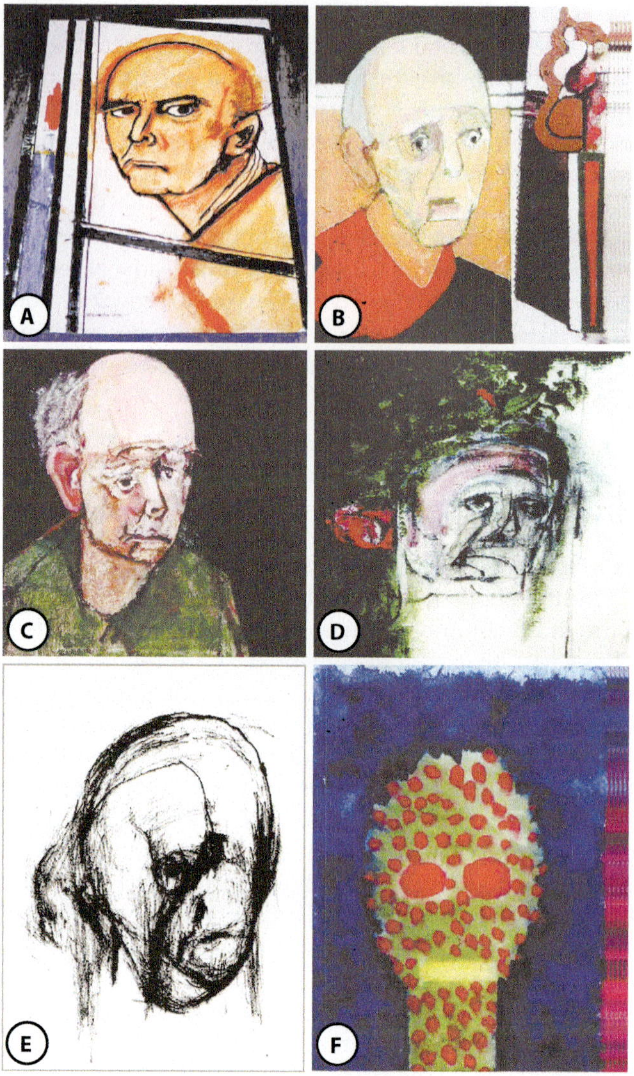

FIGS. 1A TO F: Utermohlen's deteriorating self-portraits with advancement of his Alzheimer's disease (AD).

investigations, mostly to exclude any treatable forms of dementia, were negative. A CT scan of the brain showed diffuse cortical atrophy without any evidence of lateralized atrophy. A provisional diagnosis of AD was made. She remained withdrawn and occasionally incontinent.

About 4 years after the onset of her symptoms, her caregivers (daughters) provided her with some art papers, paints, and paint brushes basically to keep her somewhat occupied. Interestingly, she started painting beautiful paintings somewhat impulsively and would object to if someone would have tried to distract her while she had been with her paints and brushes. She appeared to be

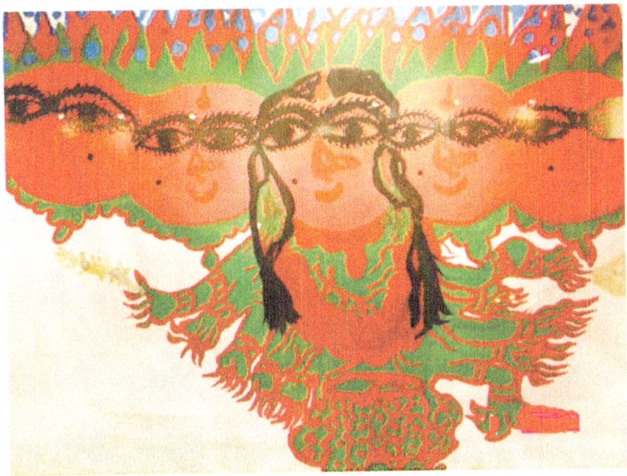

FIG. 2: Image of Goddess Durga with five heads.

very well cared for and properly attired, though it was apparent that she could not dress herself and needed help in all her daily activities of living and could only feed herself when food was placed before her. She was cheerful and greeted the author with a smile and exchanged pleasantries. Her speech was fluent without any language or semantic problems (no word finding difficulty or perseveration). She was totally disoriented in time and place. Her conversation was limited to only asking about the author's as well as his family's well-being and asking him to visit and have food in her house. Although there was no perseveration in her language, she probably had some perseveration of her thought process as she came back to the invitation issue time and again; this of course could be due to her limited vocabulary. Her comprehension for verbal and written commands was intact. She had no clue as to why and what she had been painting. She could copy with reasonable accuracy a cube, a clock face, and an overlapping pentagon. Detailed testing of her global/focal perceptual processing was not done. Her mini-mental state examination (MMSE) score[8] was 16/30 (she had 10 years school education), her clinical dementia rating scale (CDR) score[9] was 3 and activities of daily living score[10] was 12. Relative preservation of her constructional skill in the face of a low MMSE score was indeed striking. She had no focal neurological signs and her gait was normal. She was neither hypertensive nor diabetic. Her caregivers refused any further investigations including a MR brain imaging and detailed neuropsychological testing. A diagnosis of probable AD was made (NINCDS-ADRDA criteria)[11] based on clinical history, bedside cognitive function testing, and neuroimaging findings. Although the lack of detailed neuropsychological evaluation and autopsy evidence are stressed, with well-preserved language functions and the absence of any behavior disorder, the case was highly unlikely to be one of FTDs.

Her paintings were mostly of human figures, vibrant and rich in colors and with attention to details. There were many images of Hindu Gods and Goddesses (images and idols of which she must have seen several times in the past). Some of

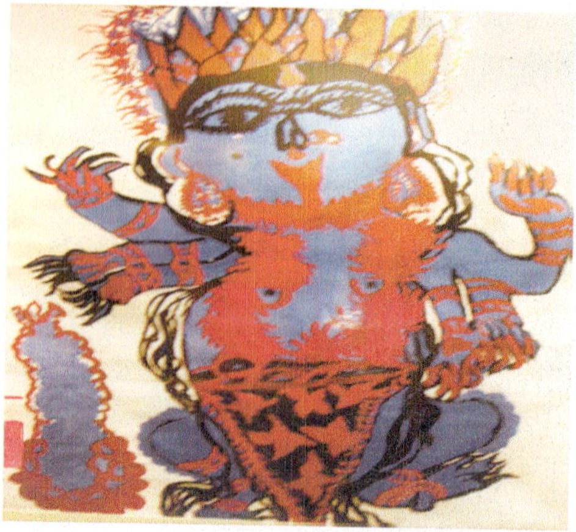

FIG. 3: Image of Goddess Kali with multiple hands.

the paintings revealed unusual multiplicity of body parts which are not generally conceived of. For example, **Figure 2** is probably of Goddess Durga as identified by her ten hands (as worshipped in Eastern India) but in the painting she has five heads. **Figure 3** probably represents Goddess Kali (dark color and protruding tongue), but drawn with multiple hands (two more than the usual four). Another painting of Kali (not reproduced here) had five heads. Such paintings of multiple body parts probably represent impulsivity and a tendency toward stereotypic activity. There were two other paintings of a very different theme—one of a girl and another of flowers. De novo development of artistic creativity in a subject with probable AD had not been recorded earlier, in contrast to patients suffering from the semantic type of frontotemporal lobar degeneration (FTLD).[4,8] The present case appeared most unlikely to be a case of FTD (especially the semantic type) because of the good preservation of language and absence of any behavioral problems.

In contrast to earlier reports,[5,6] this lady's paintings were certainly more mature, more meaningful and rich and vibrant in color and form, and certainly not abstract though somewhat unreal. The multiplicity of body parts noted in some of the paintings had been noted earlier in works of some artists with focal right hemispheric pathology (usually strokes) but not in dementias.[12] The unreality expressed in some of her paintings cannot be passed off as simply childish as she employed expert artistic techniques like "fill for space" and multilayered coloring as pointed out by the art expert. This occurred in spite of her having had no previous training in art. Many subjects with AD can easily get access to painting materials but seldom would one paint so compulsively as the present case.

What may be the possible neurocognitive basis for the emergence of de novo artistic creativity in this lady with probable AD? Any creative work needs the participation of both the cerebral hemispheres—hemispheric harmony rather than dichotomy.[13,14] Artistic creativity would be no exception. However, only clinical studies suggest that damage to the nondominant posterior parietal region severely impairs a person's artistic ability. This leads to the notion that artistic creativity is very closely linked to the functioning of the nondominant posterior parietal region—the inferior parietal lobule or sulcal area.[4,15] Based on this, it had been postulated earlier that this artistic creativity is "released" in subjects with a predominantly dominant hemisphere pathology like semantic dementia (FTD).[4] This is in conformity with the concept of "paradoxical functional facilitation" described previously[16] or the concept of "reverse diaschisis", proposed more recently.[14] The concept of lateralized compromise and release of latent creativity is purely hypothetical. This is entirely based on observations made on few isolated cases. However, Seely et al.[15] more recent publication on transmodal creativity probably provides some anatomical-physiological support to this concept. Moreover, this phenomenon is not just limited in the field of visual art, but had been observed in fields of music and literature as well.[2] On the other hand, this hemispheric model is undoubtedly a simplification. Lythgoe et al.[17] reported on a patient who, in contrast to FTD patients, developed a prolific visual artistic output in the context of a preserved language function which also enabled a prolific written poetic output. The subject had bilateral middle cerebral artery aneurysms. Conversely, Drago et al.[18] reported on an artist with Parkinson's disease whose artistic qualities significantly deteriorated following left subthalamic nucleus (STN)-deep brain stimulation (DBS), suggesting a role of the dominant hemisphere in art production which may be more than simply a deficit of motor executive function. The problem certainly is more complex in patients with bihemispheric dysfunction. The contribution of both hemispheres in creative cognition as exampled in split-brain subjects with incomplete surgical creativity in these subjects[19] probably because they cannot transmit nonverbal or emotive signals from one hemisphere to the other. This certainly is not the case here as the callosum is not generally involved by AD pathology.

The concept of lateralized compromise and facilitation does not apparently explain the de novo development of artistic creativity in this lady's case with AD where the pathology is more diffuse and more posterior than in FTD. It is hypothesized that she was premorbidly more gifted on visual abilities (which were not manifested earlier) and that her nondominant parietal lobe had been relatively spared by AD pathology, though this could not be demonstrated anatomically in the CT image. Asymmetrical cerebral involvement is known to occur in AD. It is possible that degeneration in other parts of her brain especially in the dominant hemisphere had been able to release or unmask the "hidden" artistic talents dependent on her nondominant parietal region. It is also possible that bihemispheric dysfunction in AD, by some unknown mechanism, unmasked the patient's hidden artistic talents. In this way, an analogy may be drawn between the present case and Lythgoe et al.[17] case with bilateral middle cerebral artery aneurysms and also perhaps with De Kooning's case who made some of his best paintings during his morbid years.[5]

To summarize, the exact mechanism contributing to the prolific artistic creativity in the present case remains a mystery. The question why this phenomenon is not observed in many patients with AD remains also unanswered.

ART IN FRONTOTEMPORAL DEMENTIA INCLUDING DEVELOPMENT OF DE NOVO ARTISTRY

Frontotemporal dementia seems to confer an obsessive element to artistic production characterized by the repetition of an object or pattern. Drawings and paintings retain spatial organization and proportion.

Subsequently drawings became increasingly distorted, alien, and lacking in emotion. Artists appear to develop a more realistic style with a focus on content and accuracy.

Current interest in the subject of emergent artistic skills was kindled in 1996, when Miller et al.[20] reported that a patient with FTD had developed startling new artistic creativity in the face of advancing dementia. They described a 68-year-old male with a 12-year history of FTD, who, at the age of 56 years, started to paint having had no previous interest in art. Over the next decade, he drew with increasing precision. Miller et al.[21] later included their first patient again, and described four more patients who developed new artistic skills among 69 patients with FTLD. All five patients had taken up artistic activities: three took up painting, one took up photography, and one took up small-scale sculpture, and it was noted that patients became intensely preoccupied with their art (compulsivity).

Liu et al., in 2009, described a 53-year-old, right-handed man with a history of bipolar disorder who presented with language and behavior impairments characteristic of FTLD, then developed motor symptoms consistent with a second diagnosis of amyotrophic latera sclerosis. Though the patient had never created visual art before, he developed a compulsion for painting beginning at the earliest stages of his disease, and continued producing art daily until he could no longer lift a paint brush because of his motor deficits. Upon autopsy, he was found to have ubiquitin and TDP43-positive inclusions with MND pathology.

What may be the neural mechanisms involved art production in FTD? Neuronal loss in the frontal and anterior temporal cortex in FTD may result in a change in personality, emotional blunting, lack of empathy, and perseverative behavior (Lund and Manchester Groups, 1994). All of these changes can be identified in the artworks of artists and nonartists with FTD.

The repetitive, obsessional aspects of the art may be linked to frontal executive disinhibition. Empathy and emotional blunting may be caused by orbitofrontal or temporal amygdala involvement especially in the right hemisphere (Mendez and Perryman, 2003) and perhaps not due to any involvement of the posterior temporal face processing area as occurs in AD.

The relative sparing of parietal and occipital cortex results in intact visual perceptual aspects of the art (color, contrast, spatial, etc.).

Similarly, the change in use of color in FTD is unlikely to reflect pathology in color-specialized cortex as color naming is generally intact (Robinson and Cipolotti, 2001) and the anterior distribution of atrophy is likely to spare posterior temporo-occipital cortex (area V4) specialized for color. Such artists often choose the same color persistently throughout one painting suggesting the role of frontal perseveration rather than a defect in color perception.

A number of studies, as stated earlier, have reported enhanced creativity or de novo development of artistic creativity in FTD patients.[4,20-22] But this is not universal as cases with poor or deteriorating artistic skills have also been reported[3] probably suggesting that integrity of the frontal cortex may be needed for creative processes. The exact mechanism of increased creativity or de novo artistry is not clear. It may be due to the phenomenon of "paradoxical functional facilitation" discussed earlier in relation to AD. But, perhaps, it is more likely due to the release of involuntary behaviors resulting in compulsive and disinhibited artistic output. It may be that the apparent appearance of new artistic ability is simply the result of a lack of deterioration in some functions combined with obsessive, repeated output.

TRANSMODAL CREATIVITY

In 2009, Liu et al.[22] described the case of Anne Adams who was born in 1940 and started painting architectural buildings in water color at the age of 35 years. Soon over the next 6 years, she developed an impulsiveness to paint and painted a large number of paintings of similar nature. Over the years, her painting style and subjects changed and when of 52 years of age, she was painting vibrant colorful ones of nature. At the same time, she acquired the skill to transform to visual forms and painted two symphonies named "*Rondo alla Turca*" and "*Rhapsody in Blue*". One year later, she painted the famous symphony Bolero conducted by the greatest French musician Maurice Ravel with the help of colored vertical bands which represented the various components of the music. It looked like rows of colored flags hanging side by side **(Fig. 4)**.

By the age of 58, she was painting abstracts and a period of intense creativity followed. Among her works at this time was painting the Greek symbol Pi. At the age of 60 years, she started having progressive difficulty with her speech which would fit in with a clinical diagnosis primary progressive aphasia (PPA). At 64 years of age, she was totally mute. She died in 2007 aged 67 years. Autopsy

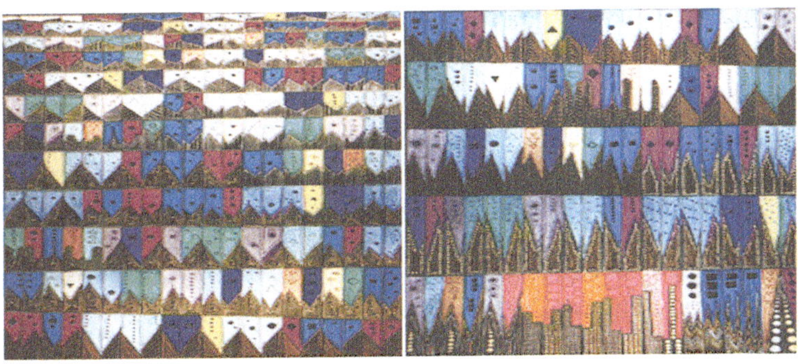

FIG. 4: Anne Adams' painting of Bolero.

and Voxel-based morphometry revealed severe atrophy of the left frontal lobe (accounting for the progressive aphasia) and increased gray matter in the right intraparietal sulcal region, possibly accounting for her artistic talents. Histology revealed Tau pathology and final diagnosis had been corticobasal degeneration. This case illustrates the rare phenomenon of transmodal creativity where auditory stimulation could be transformed into visual artistic creativity. Interestingly, Maurice Ravel (1875–1937) died of a similar disease and examined by the famous French neurologist Gilles de la Tourette.

The present author saw, in 2014, a 71 years celebrated professional artist with moderately advanced Parkinson's disease who was intolerant to levodopa to start with but later could be stabilized. He continued to paint and there was no change in his style nor any evidence of impulsivity. He published a book where he painted images on the themes of poems composed by famous poets and men of literature **(Figs. 5A to C)**.

By mid-2015, he had rapid deterioration in his motor functions and was soon bed bound and developed dysphasia and incontinence. The speech defect progressed and he was unable to recognize people. When he attempted to paint, he had visuospatial problem with moving the brush much away from the canvas. A provisional diffuse Lewy body disease was made. The question remains—did this artist also exhibited transmodal creativity with literary stimuli being transformed into his visual artistic creativity. Leonardo da Vinci rightly wrote *"Painting is poetry that is seen rather than felt, and poetry is painting that is felt rather than seen"*.

ART IN DIFFUSE LEWY BODY DISEASE

Mervyn Laurence Peake (1911–1968) was an English writer, artist, poet, and illustrator. In the last 8 years of his life, he was showing unmistakable early symptoms of dementia, for which he was given electroconvulsive therapy, to little avail. Over the next few years, he gradually lost the ability to draw steadily and quickly, although he still managed to produce some drawings with the help of his wife. Clinical features with prominent visual hallucinations suggested the diagnosis of Lewy body dementia. His later works, compared to his premorbid sketches, show dramatic loss of detail, caricature like representations and simplification. It had been suggested that the content of these later works may had been influenced by visual hallucinations. Twisted figures and beasts often appeared in Mervyn Peake's premorbid drawings, there was no dearth of these in his later sketches also.[23] In 2006, Drago et al.[24] described a patient in whom initially realistic style progressed to more abstract representation. Patients with DLB perform worse than AD patients on tests involving color-related visual tasks, pentagon copying, and have lesser degree of occipitotemporal activation on face processing tasks.

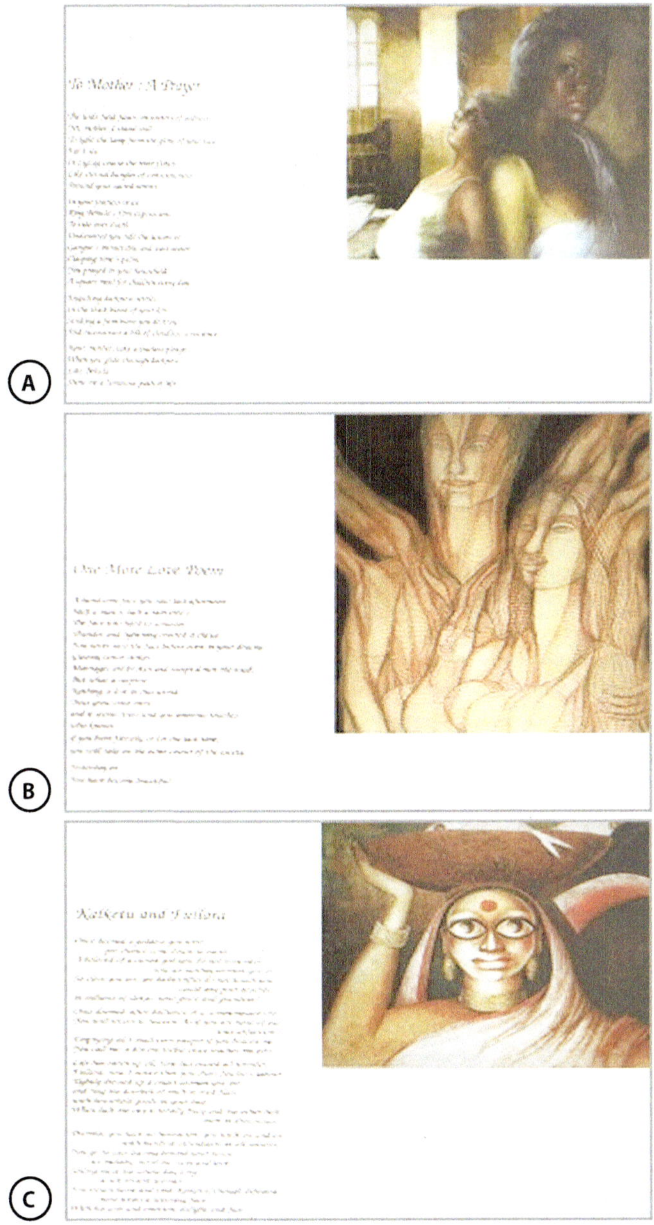

FIGS. 5A TO C: A page from the artist's book, featuring poems alongside the corresponding painting.

CONCLUDING REMARKS

There indeed are broad differences in visual perceptual aspects of the art of AD, FTD, and DLB patients. In AD, the predominant change is spatial; in DLB, all visual perceptual functions are affected; and in FTD, artworks are marked by the use of perseverative themes and a shift to realistic representation. These findings differ from those described in nonartists,[3] perhaps because the impact of dementia on art production is different in someone with extensive training and highly developed artistic skills compared with someone with only limited experience.

REFERENCES

1. Gretton C, Ffytche DH. Art and the brain: a view from dementia. Int J Geriatr Psychiatry. 2014;29(2):111-26.
2. Pollak TA, Mulvenna CM, Lythgoe M. De novo artistic behavior following brain injury. In: Bogouselavsky J, Hennerici MG (Eds). Neurological Disorders in Famous Artists (Part 2). Basel: Karger; 2007. pp. 75-88.
3. Rankin KP, Liu AA, Howard S, Slama H, Hou CE, Shuster K, et al. A case controlled study of altered visual art production in Alzheimer's and FTLD. Cogn Behav Neurol. 2007;20:48-61.
4. Miller BL, Hou CE. Portraits of artists. Emergence of visual creativity in dementia. Arch Neurol. 2004;61:842-4.
5. Espinel CH. Memory and creation of Art: The syndrome, as in de Kooning of creating in the midst of dementia. In: Bogousslavsky J, Hennerici MG (Eds). Neurological Disorders in Famous Artists (Part 2). Basel: Karger; 2007. pp. 150-68.
6. Cummings JL, Zarit JM. Probable Alzheimer's disease in an artist. JAMA. 1987;258:2731-4.
7. Crutch SJ, Issacs R, Rossor MN. Some workmen can blame their tools: Artistic change in an individual with Alzheimer's disease. Lancet. 2001;357:2129-33.
8. Folstein MF, Folstein SE, McHugh PR. "Mini-mental state". A practical method for grading the mental state of patients for the clinician. J Psychiatr Res. 1975;12:189-98.
9. Berg L. Clinical Dementia Rating Scale. Psychopharm Bull. 1985;24:637-9.
10. Fillenbaum GG. Activities of Daily Living and Instrumental Activities of Daily Living screening in elderly. J Am Geriatr Soc. 1985;33:698-706.
11. McKhann G, Drachman D, Folstein M, Katzman R, Price D, Stadlan EM. Clinical diagnosis of Alzheimer's disease: Report of the NINCDS–ADRDA work group under the auspices of Department of Health and Human Services Task Force on Alzheimer's Disease. Neurology. 1984;34:939-44.
12. Chatterjee A. The neuropsychology of visual artistic production. Neuropsychologia. 2004;42:1568-83.
13. Heilman KM, Nadeau SE, Beversdorf DQ. Creative innovation: Possible brain mechanism. Neurocase. 2003;9:369-79.
14. Chakravarty A. The creative brain: Revisiting concepts. Med Hypotheses. 2010;74:606-12.
15. Seeley WW, Mathews BR, Richard K, Gorno-Tempini MC, Foti D, Mackenzie IR, et al. Unravelling Bolero: Progressive aphasia, transmodal creativity and the right posterior neocortex. Brain. 2008;131:39-49.
16. Kapur N. Paradoxical functional facilitation in brain – behavior research. A critical review. Brain. 1996;119:1775-90.
17. Lythgoe MF, Pollak TA, Kalmus M, De Hann M, Chong WK. Obsessive, prolific artistic output following subarachnoid hemorrhage. Neurology. 2005;64:397-8.
18. Drago V, Foster PS, Okun MS, Cosentino FI, Conigliaro R, Haq I, et al. Turning off artistic ability: The influence of left DBS in art production. J Neurol Sci. 2009;281:116-21.

19. Gazzaniga MS. Consciousness and the cerebral hemisphere. In: Gazzaniga MS (Ed). The Cognitive Neurosciences. Cambridge, Massachusetts: MIT Press; 1995. pp. 1391-404.
20. Miller BL, Ponton M, Benson DF, Cummings JL, Mena I. Enhanced artistic creativity with temporal lobe degeneration. Lancet. 1996;348:1744-5.
21. Miller BL, Cummings J, Mishkin F, Boone K, Prince F, Ponton M, et al. Emergence of artistic talent in frontotemporal dementia. Neurology. 1998;51:978-82.
22. Liu A, Werner K, Roy S, Trojanowski JQ, Morgan-Kane U, Miller BL, et al. A case study of an emerging visual artist with frontotemporal lobar degeneration and amyotrophic lateral sclerosis. Neurocase. 2009;15:235-47.
23. Sahlas DJ. Dementia with Lewy bodies and the neurobehavioral decline of Mervyn Peake. Arch Neurol. 2003;60:889-92.
24. Drago V, Crucian GP, Foster PS, Cheong J, Finney GR, Pisani F, et al. Lewy body dementia and creativity: case report. Neuropsychologia. 2006;44:3011-5.

CHAPTER

11

Artistic Talent in Dyslexia: A Hypothesis

INTRODUCTION: HOW DID IT ALL BEGIN?

In late December 2007, a Hindi movie named Taare Zameen Par (Stars on Earth) was released in India directed by the famous actor Aamir Khan. The film was a box-office hit. The film portrayed the tormented life of a young boy who could not read or write properly. He was bullied at school as well as at home by his parents. This continued until he met his new art teacher at the boarding school who diagnosed his dyslexia.

The art teacher also noted some hidden visual artistic skill in the boy. With the teacher's guidance and encouragement, the boy excelled in painting and won the school painting competition.

The film had a happy ending. Having watched the movie twice, I simply marveled at the theme and wondered if it was only the script writer's fantasy or there was science behind it and there began my research.

LEARNING DISABILITIES: AN OVERVIEW

Learning refers to the higher and most complex cognitive function of the brain and it should be of no surprise that many children (as many as 5% worldwide) have problems acquiring the basics of reading, writing, and mathematics. Many children in first and second grade just need some more time to acquire these basic skills. These temporary learning problems are frequent and reflect normal maturational variability. At the end of the continuous spectrum (and hence an arbitrary cut off is to be used), however, there are children who really have fundamental and persistent learning problems. They are learning disabled.[1] A learning disability is usually defined as an unexpected, specific, and persistent failure to acquire efficient academic skills despite conventional instruction, and adequate intelligence and sociocultural opportunity.[2] Although all fields in learning can be affected, it seems that learning problems can be classified into one of two major categories. The largest group of children has problems with language skills, in reading and spelling: The dyslexia group or the basic phonologic processing disabilities.

The other group of children has more problems with problem solving, with arithmetic and visuospatial problems and with motor and tactile perceptual problems. These children are classified within the large group of nonverbal learning disabilities. It comprises the group of children with dyscalculia. Perhaps, one of the most intriguing observations is the fact that children in both groups also show cognitive strengths. Many children in dyslexia group show relative proficiencies in problem solving and in visuospatial skills. These two features highlight the normal intelligence in most dyslexic children and their artistic talents.

Identified by Oswald Berkhan in 1881,[3] the term "dyslexia" was later coined in 1887 by Rudolf Berlin, an ophthalmologist practicing in Stuttgart, Germany.[4] He used the term to refer to a case of a young boy who had a severe impairment in learning to read and write in spite of showing typical intellectual and physical abilities in all other aspects.

The advent of neuroimaging techniques to study brain structure and function enhanced the research in the 1980s and 1990s. Since then, interest in the neurologically based causes persisted.

Current models of the relation between the brain and dyslexia generally focus on some form of defective or delayed maturation of brain. More recently, genetic research has provided increasing evidence supporting a genetic origin of dyslexia. Researchers are searching for a link between the neurological and genetic findings and the reading disorder. There are many previous and current theories of dyslexia, but one, that has much support from research, is that, whatever the biological cause, dyslexia is a matter of reduced phonological awareness, the ability to analyze and line units of spoken and written languages.[5] A Hong Kong study has recently shown using functional magnetic resonance imaging (fMRI) technology that the children reading English (an alphabetic language) used a different part of the brain than those reading Chinese (a nonalphabetic language).[6] Positron emission tomography (PET) and fMRI studies have produced clear evidence of structural differences in the brains of children with reading difficulties.

Dyslexic children have a deficit in parts of the dominant hemisphere (usually the left) in the inferior frontal gyrus, inferior parietal lobule, and middle and ventral temporal cortices.[7,8]

Furthermore, autopsied and neuroimaging studies suggest that dyslexic brains are usually symmetric compared to the asymmetric brains in normal children,[9] who had large left hemisphere (dominant hemisphere). Earlier, microscopic studies revealed presence of ectopias and microgyria in the inferior frontal and temporal cortices of dyslexic brains.[10] However, all children with dyslexia do not have these changes but these studies suggest some anatomical correlation of the functional disability.[11]

The dyslexia writing is characterized by spelling errors, letter order errors, letter addition/subtraction, and a small written vocabulary. The writing speed is slow, handwriting poor with irregularly formed letters and inappropriate use of words is common.

Reading at times is a near impossibility and often with highly phonetized spelling ("shud" for "should") with difficulty in distinguishing among homophones ("their" and "there").

Dyslexics occasionally have poor motor skills with poor coordination and clumsiness. Dyslexia, as indicated earlier, should not be confused with dyscalculia and, in fact, dyslexic individuals can be gifted in mathematics (e.g., Albert Einstein). However, descriptive mathematics, engineering or physics problems that relay on written texts rather than numbers may pose problem (exception Leonardo da Vinci and Einstein). Also, there may be difficulty remembering mathematical facts, such as multiplication tables, and learning the sequence of steps when performing calculations. Response to mathematic drills is often slow. It is important to realize at this stage that the disability in learning disorders is often domain specific (just like intelligence) and all affected individuals may not manifest all features detailed above. Specific brain regions or specific circuitry performs specific functions, the details of which have not yet been unraveled.

ARTISTIC CREATIVITY AND DYSLEXIA

Dyslexic people often have a natural flair for one or more of the arts such as music, dance, drawing, or acting. Dyslexic people also often possess a natural ability to see patterns in noise, producing creative abstract ideas pulled out of what many would look upon as mundane sensory environments.[12]

Leonardo da Vinci (1452–1519) is one of the greatest creative artists the world has ever seen. He painted such masterpieces as the Mona Lisa, The Madonna and Child, Leda and the Swan, and many others. But he also excelled as an engineer (planned and sketched an entire canal system in ancient Italy and designed bridges), an architect (architectural plan of churches), and made in-depth excellent drawings of human anatomy including two showing the anatomy of human sexual intercourse. From a detailed study of his writing, it has been suggested that Leonardo might have had dyslexia.[13] Story goes that Picasso also learnt to read and write late. So, he could also have developmental learning disorder. Back in 1977, Cohn and Neumann,[12] in a study of dyslexic children, observed that some have an outstanding ability to produce artistic pictures and objects. These productions were perceptive, well organized, and generally contained much action.

Despite these pictorial skills, these patients might have only a rudimentary use of coded symbolic graphic forms. These workers postulated for the first time that artistic production is generated by the nondominant hemisphere and that this function is quite distinct from the coded graphic operation resident in the dominant hemisphere (to be discussed later in this article). In a more recent study,[14] it has been found that art academy students reported significantly more signs of dyslexia than nonart university students. Objective testing showed poorer phonological skills among art students. The incidence of dyslexia was far higher among art students.

CREATIVITY IN DYSLEXIA: LESSON FROM EINSTEIN'S BRAIN

Albert Einstein (1879–1955) is undoubtedly one of the greatest creative geniuses of modern times. As a child, he started talking late and researchers later learnt that he had developmental dyslexia (DD). Einstein's own description[15] of his scientific thinking was that "...words do not seem to play any role", but there is "associative play" of "more of less clear images" of a "visual and muscular ideation". He himself recognized that a useful method for understanding brain's role in creativity would be to study the brains of highly creative people. He willed that his brain be removed before cremation and be studied in detail for medical research. This was done in 1955 (when he died of ruptured aortic aneurysm) and the brain was fixed and photographed and studied both macroscopically and microscopically (although out of the 240 pieces in which it was cut most got lost). Macroscopically, the exceptional finding had been that in Einstein's brain, the stem of the lateral sulcus was found to be continuous with the bottom end of the postcentral sulcus.[16] This is in contrast to usual anatomy where the posterior ramus of the lateral sulcus goes beyond the postcentral sulcus into the parietal lobe on which lies the supramarginal gyrus, the angular gyrus lies behind it and the two constitute the Wernicke's area. These two gyri together with the part of parietal lobe lying below the intraparietal sulcus constitute the inferior parietal lobule corresponding to Brodmann's areas 39 and 40. The peculiar anatomical variation in Einstein's brain resulted in a large undivided inferior parietal lobule (areas 39 and 40). The inferior parietal lobule, especially in the nondominant hemisphere, is the seat of visuospatial cognition, mathematical ideation, and imagery movement as also of artistic and literal creativity.[17,18] In Einstein's brain, as a result of the altered sulcal anatomy, this area was larger than controls and remained undivided allowing for uninterrupted connectivity. Histological study by Diamond and others[19] earlier indicated that Einstein's area 39 showed a lesser number of neurons but proportionately a higher number of glial cells. This was later interpreted as suggestive of greater connectivity[20] and his mathematical genius thus seemed related to his large undivided inferior parietal lobule (areas 39 and 40) and greater connectivity in this region. In 1985, Geschwind and Galaburda[21] posited that delay in development of the left hemisphere (dominant) may allow the right hemisphere (nondominant) which mediates spatial computing to become highly specialized. It can thus be postulated that Einstein's DD, causally related to a developmental delay of the dominant hemisphere, might have led to the nondominant hemisphere being highly specialized for spatial computation.

This hypothesis seems a sound one but difficult to prove and fail to explain why all dyslexic children do not become as creative as Einstein. Neurological outcome from localized brain injury is extremely individualized. Lot depends on plasticity and connectivity.

ARTISTIC CREATIVITY AND NEUROLOGICAL DISORDERS

Like visuospatial cognition, artistic creativity most likely rests in the parietal lobe (especially the nondominant one) and more so in the inferior parietal lobar region. It is supposed that normally the dominant hemisphere has an inhibitory influence on creative (especially artistic and literal) functions on the nondominant parietal lobe. Does that mean that "disinhibition" of the nondominant parietal lobe from a dominant hemisphere lesion would increase artistic and literary creativity?

Up until now, there are a number of reports of de novo development of artistic behavior following brain injury especially affecting the dominant hemisphere.[22] Such pathologies include left temporal lobe epileptic focus, dominant hemisphere stroke, subarachnoid hemorrhage caused by middle cerebral aneurysm, and most importantly frontotemporal dementia where dominant hemisphere affection with language disorder is well recognized. These case histories support the notion that a dominant hemispheric dysfunction may lead to "disinhibited" functioning of the nondominant parietal lobe to result in unmasking of hidden artistic talent a phenomenon described much earlier by Kapur[23] and called "paradoxical functional facilitation". This he thought, as a compensatory augmentation occurring as a specific manifestation of central nervous system (CNS) plasticity. Likewise, hypergraphia may result from dominant hemispheric injury but this would not be discussed here.

ARTISTIC TALENT IN DYSLEXIA: A HYPOTHESIS

Based on the arguments relating creativity to dyslexia as in Einstein's case and de novo development of artistic creativity in dominant hemispheric brain-injured patients, it can now be hypothesized, at this stage, that unmasking or development of artistic talents observed in many dyslexic subjects (vide supra) may be linked to the developmental delay in language function localized in the dominant hemisphere (usually left hemisphere).

This would "disinhibit" the nondominant parietal lobe (usually the right) to unmask or develop artistic talents and creativity. Creativity of course is domain specific and it need not be limited only in the field of art.

In support of this hypothesis that underfunctioning of one part of brain may lead to disinhibited functioning of another part unmasking a skill or talent, are the cases where artistic talents have been recognized in children with autism spectrum disorders,[24] which fundamentally result from a developmental underconnectivity in the brain.[25] In the light of the proposed hypothesis, it seems justified to say that, in autism, underconnectivity in one part of brain facilitates development of functional hyperconnectivity in another part unmasking talents. Such talented autistic patients are often referred to as autistic savants.[26,27] The literal meaning of the word "savant" is "scholar". I feel that dyslexic child with exceptional artistic or other talents may also be referred to as "dyslexic savants".

RECENT OBSERVATIONS

Mastering the phonological principle is essential for all reading, hence failure to do so cannot be used to distinguish developmental dyslexia (DD) from the many other causes of such failure. Thus, many new psychological, signal detection, and neurological theories have been introduced recently. All suggest the idea that DD is fundamentally caused by impaired signaling of the timing of the visual and auditory cues that are essential for reading. At the cellular level, large "magnocellular" neurons which respond rapidly to sensory transients seem to the principal culprit. Of much interest are intervention studies that have shown that improving magnocellular function improves dyslexic children's reading, together with cohort studies that have demonstrated that the magnocellular timing deficit is present in infants who later become dyslexic, long before they begin learning to read. Conversely, it may be possible that dyslexic children gain parvocellular abundance to compensate for magnocellular deficit.[28] This may often impart the exceptional "holistic" talents that have been ascribed to them and that society needs to nurture.

CONCLUDING REMARKS

If the hypotheses proposed in the article are correct, it would seem socially beneficial to allow children with dyslexia to develop their unique artistic ability (or other skills) to its full capacity and not to overemphasize the correction of the disturbed coded symbol operations, in remedial training.

REFERENCES

1. Shatwitz SE, Gruen JR, Shaywitz BA. Management of dyslexia, its rationale and underlying neurobiology. Pediatr Clin North Am. 2007;54:609-23.
2. Shaywitz SE. Dyslexia. N Engl J Med. 1998;338:307-12.
3. Wikipedia. Oswald Berkhan (19 March 1834 – 15 February 1917). [online] Available from https://en.wikipedia.org/wiki/Oswald_Berkhan. [Last accessed February, 2025]
4. Berlin R. Uber dyslexia. Archiv Fur Psychiatry. 1887;15:276-8.
5. Lyytinen H, Erskine J, Mikko A, Richardson U. Reading and reading disorders. In: Blackwell Hand Book of Language Development. London: Blackwell; 2007. pp. 454-74.
6. Siok WT, Niu Z, Jin Z, Perfetti CA, Tan LH. A structural functional basis for dyslexia in the cortex of Chinese readers. Proc Nat Acad Sci USA. 2008;105:5561-5.
7. Cao F, Bitan T, Chou TL, Burman DD, Both JR. Deficient orthographic and phonological representations in children with dyslexia revealed by brain activation patterns. J Child Psychol Psychiatry. 2006;47:1041-50.
8. Shaywitz BA, Lyon GR, Shaywitz SE. The role of functional magnetic resonance imaging in understanding reading and dyslexia. Dev Neuropsychol. 2006;30:613-32.
9. Haslam R, Dalby JT, Hohns RD, Rademaker AM. Cerebral asymmetry in developmental dyslexia. Arch Neurol. 1981;27:23-5.
10. Galaburda AM, Kemper TL. Cytoarchitectonic abnormalities in developmental dyslexia: a case study. Ann Neurol. 1979;6:94-100.
11. Sherman G. Can neuroscience help to demystify dyslexia. UK: Schwab Learning; 2007.
12. Cohn R, Neumann MA. Artistic production in dyslectic children. Neurol Neurochir Psiquiatr. 1977;18:65-9.
13. Rosstad A. Leonardo da Vinci – a dyslectic genius? Tidsskr Nor Laegeforen. 2002;122: 2887-90.
14. Wolff U, Lundberg I. The prevalence of dyslexia among art students. Dyslexia. 2002;8:34-42.
15. Einstein A, Hadamard J. The psychology of invention in the mathematical field. New Jersey: Princeton University Press; 1949. pp. 142-3.
16. Witelson SF, Kigar DL, Harvey T. The exceptional brain of Albert Einstein. Lancet. 1999;353:2149-53.
17. Critchley M. The Parietal Lobes. New York: Hafner Publications; 1971.
18. Miller BL. Creativity in the context of neurological illness. CNS Spectr. 2008;13:7-9.
19. Diamond MC, Scheibel AB, Murphy Jr GH, Harvey T. On the brain of a scientist: Albert Einstein. Exp Neurol. 1985;88:198-204.
20. Heilman KM, Nadeaeu SE, Beversdorf DO. Creative innovation: possible brain mechanisms. Neurocase. 2003;9:369-79.

21. Geschwind N, Galaburda AM. Cerebral lateralization. Biological mechanisms, associations and pathology: III. A hypothesis and program for research. Arch Neurol. 1985;42(7):634-54.
22. Pollak TA, Mulvenna CM, Lythgoe MF. De novo artistic behavior following brain injury. In: Bogousslavsky J, Hennerici MG (Eds). Neurological Disorders in Famous Artists – Part 2, volume 22. Basel: Karger; 2007. pp. 75-88.
23. Kapur N. Paradoxical functional facilitation in brain-behavior research. A critical review. Brain. 1996;119:1775-90.
24. Selfe L. Nadia: A Case of Extraordinary Drawing Ability in an Autistic Child. New York: Academic Press; 1977.
25. Deelay Q, Murphy D. Pathophysiology of autism: evidence from brain imaging. Br J Hosp Med (London). 2009;70:138-42.
26. Hou C, Miller BL, Cummings JL, Goldberg M, Mychack P, Bottino V, et al. Autistic savants. Neuropsychiatry Neuropsychol Behav Neurol. 2000;13(1):29-38.
27. Takahata K, Kato M. Neural mechanism underlying autistic savant and acquired savant syndrome. Brain Nerve. 2008;60:861-9.
28. Stein J. Theories about developmental dyslexia. Brain Sci. 2023;13(2):208.

(Reprinted with modifications from Chakravarty A. Artistic talent in dyslexia—a hypothesis. Med Hypotheses. 2009;73(4):569-71.)

COMMENTARY

A Brief Note on Autistic Art

Ambar Chakravarty

Let me start with a quiz. The picture below shows two horses. Which one do you think is a better drawing? The one on your right of course. You would be surprised to learn that the one on your left had been one drawn by none other than Leonardo da Vinci while the one on the right had been the work of a 17-year-old autistic child from Poland who was brought up in the United States. The girl's creativity exceeded that of da Vinci at least in this drawing **(Fig. 1)**.

Such heightened creativity in children with autism spectrum disorders (ASDs) is not too uncommon. In Nadia's case with improvement in her autistic behavior with appropriate training, her artistic creativity had been on the wane. Truly speaking, Leonardo's sketch has more dynamism (speed of galloping) in it as evidenced by the positions of the horse's legs and the positions of its hoofs (angular rather than flat as in case of Nadia's sketch).

Autism spectrum disorder comprises neurological and developmental disorders that affect interaction of one individual with others, interpersonal communication, learning, and behavior. Symptoms generally appear in the first

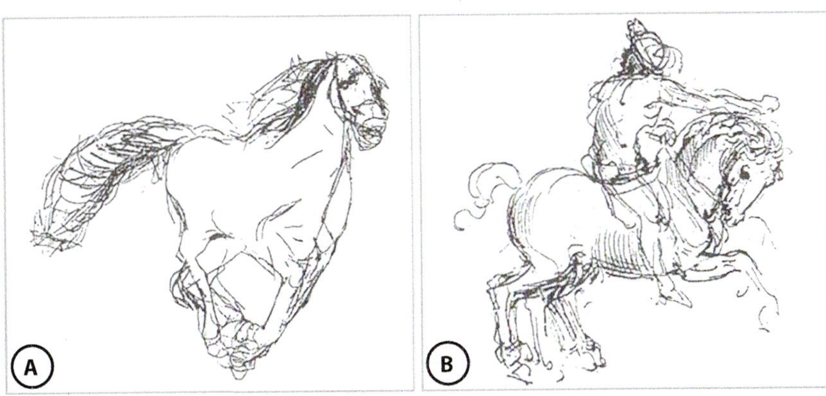

FIGS. 1A AND B: Comparison of horse drawings.

2 years of life, but diagnosis is often delayed and autism can be diagnosed at any age. Hence, it is described as a "developmental disorder".

According to the *Diagnostic and Statistical Manual of Mental Disorders (DSM-5)*, of the American Psychiatric Association, people with ASD often have:

- Difficulty with communication and interaction with other people
- Restricted interests and repetitive behaviors
- Symptoms that affect their ability to function in school, work, and other areas of life

The primary causes of ASD are not known, but studies suggest that both genetic and environmental factors play together to affect development in ways that lead to ASD. Conceptually, it may be suggested that there occurs some developmental abnormality in the speech area connections in the dominant hemisphere, while dyslexia develops when there occurs a delay in development of these connecting pathways. Artistic creativity in both autism and dyslexia may have the same conceptual mechanism, namely a disinhibition of the dominant hemispheric functions over the nondominant hemisphere's role in artistic production.

Autistic artists with better linguistic and communication skills often show more originality and attention to detail than their nonautistic counterparts, with a positive correlation between artistic talent and *high linguistic functioning.*[1,2] Autistic art is often considered *outsider art.*[3] The works of some autistic artists, however, have featured in art publications and documentaries and been exhibited in mainstream galleries. Although autistic artists seldom received formal *art education* in the past, recently facilities for formal training of such individuals have been made available in some western countries.[4]

Some degree of eccentricity used to be regarded as just a part of the artistic personality. Nowadays, the possibility that this was due to some kind of personality disorder is usually considered. Psychologists often suggested some mild form of high functioning autism, like Asperger's syndrome in some autistic artists. Interestingly, when highly gifted people with mild form of autism show artistic ability, the arts they produce have a distinctive character termed "The beautiful otherness of the autistic mind".[5]

REFERENCES

1. Pennisi P, Giallongo L, Milintenda G, Cannarozzo M. Autism, autistic traits and creativity: a systematic review and meta-analysis. Cogn Process. 2021;22(4):733.
2. Baron-Cohen S, Ashwin E, Ashwin C, Tavassoli T, Chakrabarti B. Talent in autism: hyper-systemizing, hyper-attention to detail and sensory hypersensitivity. Philos Trans R Soc Lond B Biol Sci. 2009;364(1522):1377-83.
3. Autism Connect. Museums thrust autistic artists into the mainstream.
4. Wheeler M. Academic Supports for College Students with an Autism Spectrum Disorder: Articles: Indiana Resource Center for Autism: Indiana University Bloomington. [online] Available from https://www.iidc.indiana.edu/irca/articles/academic-supports-for-college-students-with-an-autism-spectrum-disorder.html. [Last accessed February, 2025]
5. Happé F, Frith U. The beautiful otherness of the autistic mind. Philos Trans R Soc Lond B Biol Sci. 2009;27;364(1522):1346-50.

CHAPTER

12

Neurology and Literature

INTRODUCTION

The principal duty of a neurologist is to protect the condition of healthy individuals and promoting adequate preventive measures and spreading knowledge of them among the population. The key features would include making the public aware of neurological diseases, their most well-known aspect being integrated care and treatment of neurological patients. Social stigmas represent one of the aspects that most seriously compromises quality of life for a patient with epilepsy being the most notorious neurological disorder. This may be due to the dramatic character of its manifestations, its atavistic demonization, but most importantly its negative social connotations and restrictions coupled with the fact that it goes unnoticed most of the times.

Fictions contribute a lucid view of neurological diseases in general and of epilepsy in particular bridging the gap between doctors and patients and also bringing readers closer to a more accessible reality, free from the complicated medical jargon. Literature may have a possible role in the professional development of neurologists by contributing concision and clarity to the expression in the words of ideas. In the words of Gregorio Maranon (1887–1960; Spanish physician, scientist, historian, writer, and philosopher)—"If we doctors were not only fond of literature, but proficient in its technique—great poets, in short—it is obvious that we would be much closer to being understood by all, and therefore closer to curing all those disorders..." Thomas Sydenham (1624–1689) (of Sydenham's chorea fame) told his disciple Richard Blackmore on what book to read to become a better doctor—"Read Don Quixote".[1] Peter Davies thinks that the poem "Do Not Go Gentle into That Good Night" by Dylan Thomas reveals more about the reactions of man to death than any textbook. The poet offers insight into how to face death with dignity and ferocity rather than resignation, believing that people should "burn and rave" as they approach death. Joao Lobo Antunes, a neurosurgeon, felt that a good doctor must have a combination of scientific knowledge and cultural awareness.[2]

FICTIONS, WRITERS, AND NEUROLOGY

The aim of practicing medicine is to provide effective treatment that is sometimes curative, often palliative, and always comforting. Three decades ago, evidence-based medicine (EBM) arose for the purpose of protecting patients and preventing unnecessary drug trials. This involves combining the doctor's own clinical skill with the best available external medical evidence, gathered by means of systematic studies. Here, decision making is based on the evidence obtained through randomized double-blind clinical trials. The doctor's skill and clinical judgement join forces with accumulated experience and common sense so that he or she can make informed decisions on how best to treat and care for the patient[3] and where possible reducing, damage arising from scientific and technological advances.

The term "narrative-based medicine" or NBM is a recent invention, although the idea was extensively described by Laín Entralgo in the middle of the past century.[4] The patient's story is critically analyzed to better understand its meaning and using the patient's symptoms or subjective descriptions of the ailments or discomforts as a basis for evaluating the objective and quantifiable findings from clinical examinations or laboratory tests. As such, the language employed should ease doctor–patient communication, rather than creating barriers in its path. Hence, discouraging terms like "untreatable" should be phased out in favor of more neutral words like "drug-resistant" in such chronic diseases as epilepsy. The same is true in cases of terminal illnesses—an example would be amyotrophic lateral sclerosis (ALS)—which has no effective cure but the patient may benefit from some degree of relief and consolation from regimens such as feeding gastrostomy and portable ventilators. In any case, the patient's own accounts will often determine the treatment protocol. In fact, there is no one better for telling the story of a disease or events in a medical history than a well-informed patient. This helps us understand the extent of the discomfort caused by the disease.

Medicine and literature should not be considered fields foreign to each other, since the relationship between doctors and writers constitutes an example of symbiosis where both disciplines have been enriched by their mutual contributions. Probably one of the most paradigmatic examples is Anton Pavlovich Chekhov, who came to affirm that medicine was his wife and literature was his lover. Other examples are François Rabelais, Arthur Conan Doyle, William Somerset Maugham, Andrés Bello, Pío Baroja, Gregorio Marañón, Laín Entralgo, Miguel Torga, Luis Pimentel, Antonio Lobo Antunes, Luis Martín Santos, Juan Antonio Vallejo Nájera, and Oliver Sacks, among others.

Oliver Sacks (1933–2015), with his view that neurological diseases are not shackles, but rather open windows from which we can observe different forms of consciousness and develop new facets and latent talents, has emerged as one of the most popular authors representing the specialty. He describes the fascinating experiences of his patients in such books as *The Man who Mistook His Wife for a Hat, Migraine, Awakenings, and An Anthropologist on Mars.* Sacks's stories are neither literary fiction nor dramatized medical histories. Rather, they constitute erudite, reflexive, and systematic presentations of interesting cases, accurately taken from his own neurological practice. In each anecdote, the patient's narrative serves as the guiding clue of the appropriate diagnosis and management.

In the specific field of neurology, fictional literature provides a lucid look at neurological diseases, building a bridge between the doctor and the patient, bringing the reader closer to a more accessible reality devoid of complex medical jargon, and contributing to establishing a meeting point in the social framework. In some cases, literary descriptions have preceded medical description, as, for example, in the captivity syndrome (locked-in syndrome), described in the work of Alexandre Dumas. The Count of Monte Cristo (1844), in which the elderly Noirtier de Villefort is immobile and uses blinking and eye movements to communicate (locked in syndrome); in Therese Raquin (1867) by Émile Zola also appears an old woman with this pathological condition. Subsequently, the dramatic symptoms of captivity syndrome have been described in the first person by Jean-Dominique Bauby in The Diving Suit and the Butterfly (1997).

Migraine

In 1955, Todd suggested the term Alice in Wonderland to define the metamorphosis generally associated with migraine inspired by deformed visual perceptions typical of the characters in the famous book by Lewis Carrol.[5] Affected subjects may experience two types of hallucinations namely visual and somesthetic (body image). An array of symptoms involving altered perception of shape (metamorphopsia) of objects or persons who appear to be smaller (micropsia) or larger (macropsia) than normal, of impaired sense of passage of time, of zooming of the environment, are often associated with depersonalization and derealization. On the whole, somesthetic hallucinations are more common than pure visual ones. The causes of the syndrome include—Epstein-Barr virus (EBV) and other viral infections including H1N1, migraine, HaNDL, epilepsy, and topiramate use.

Multiple Sclerosis

WNP Barbellion (pseudonym used by the naturalist Bruce Fredrick Cummings) gave details of his own progressive multiple sclerosis (MS) on a day-to-day basis. *The Journal of a Disappointed Man*, filled with frank and keen observation, unique philosophy, and personal resignation, was described by its author as "a study in the nude". The book received both adulatory and scathing reviews. But his account familiarized people with the same disease which ultimately led to the formation of the MS Society allover[6] the world. The author described various clinical forms of the disease including the type affecting the brainstem predominantly. Barbellion sums up his life in one of the last entries in *The Journal of a Disappointed Man*: "I am only twenty-eight, but I have telescoped into those few years a tolerably long life: I have loved and married, and have a family; I have wept and enjoyed, struggled and overcome, and when the hour comes I shall be content to die."[6]

Dementia

Alzheimer's disease is also represented in fictional literature, an example may be My Mother (2009) by Tahar Ben Jelloun, which refers to memory loss, disorientation, and personality collapse: *"The brain has begun its suicide. Personality falls apart. The millimeter wiring between cells breaks down every second. The lights run out and become intermittent".*

English writer Iris Murdoch (1919–1999) was best known for her novels about good and evil, sexual relationships, morality, and the power of the unconscious. She described problems faced by her due to Alzheimer's disease through three different novels written in three different times. The first symptom noticed by her readers had been the lack of wit compared to her previous works. It is well known that the subtility of cognition at very beginning of the illness may be missed by standard neuropsychological tests in persons with high intellect.

Rabies

Camilo Jose Sella contributed a suggestive description of human rabies in his father who was bitten by a rabid dog and had to be isolated in the pantry; "...he threw bites which would have torn an arm off anyone who had been caught; ...my father finally went quiet the following night ...and when we went to get him out, thinking he had died, we found him crouching on the floor and with such fear on his face, it seemed he had entered hell."

Neurofibromatosis

The novel "The Elephant Man", written by the London surgeon Sir Frederick Treves, is the story of a social stigmata set in the end of the 19th century that reflects both the degree of cruelty and of humanity that human beings can reach. The screenplay revolves around an ugly looking man with a large head and deformed body with multiple lumps protruding from the skin called fibromas. The condition is neurofibromatosis type 1 or Proteus syndrome caused by a genetic anomaly.

Stroke

David Lynch, who made the screenplay of the Elephant Man, also made the screenplay of the novel "The Straight Story" by Roach and Sweeney which tells the story of an elderly man who decides to cross the United States on a lawnmower to make amends with his brother to whom he had not spoken for years. The brother suffered a stroke and had dysphasia. In addition to explaining the pathophysiology of the clinical syndrome, the story makes an impression on the capacity to transform human relations.

Anton Chekhov, in Pavilion VI (1892), presents a doctor who suffers a ruptured brain aneurysm: "The next morning he woke up with a tremendous headache. He felt his whole body broken; he was immersed in an absolute morass".

Epilepsy

Writers such as Shakespeare or Cervantes have included detailed descriptions of epilepsy in their literature. The tragic plays of Shakespeare can highlight the power of emotion when it comes to causing organic disorders such as syncope and seizures; the latter being seen in cases of Julius Caesar and Othello. Cervantes, in relation to a case of epilepsy described in El Quixote, portrays a view of medicine in his time, subject to the theory of humors with bloodletting as the main therapeutic basis.

In *The Nightingale Silenced*, Anglo-Welsh writer Margiad Evans describes the treatment she underwent in a London hospital. In this book, she detailed the onset of her seizures, postictal paralysis, and the psychological damage caused by the progression of the disease. Her opinion that the cause of epilepsy as diabolical possession is an idea that probably arose among people with epilepsy themselves; those who experience seizures feel that their bodies are suddenly seized by an alien force.[3]

The British author Charles Dickens accurately describes several epileptic seizures that affect different characters in his novels, such as Monks (villain of Oliver Twist, 1839), Guster (desolate house, 1853), Anthony Chuzzlewit (life and adventures of Martin Chuzzlewit, 1844), and Bradley Heatone (our common friend, 1865).[7] In life and adventures of Martin Chuzzlewit, for example, he describes how a character suffers a grand mal crisis: "His whole appearance indicated that he was, in truth, very sick, and he shook and shook terribly, not as people do from cold, but in a horrible type of spasm or convulsion that tormented his entire body." The Pickwick Club Papers (1836–1837) describes what would later be called Pickwick syndrome, while David Copperfield (1849–1850) presents various characters with movement disorders, such as Uriah Heep, showing dyskinesias, probably due to generalized dystonia. The author mentions that the strange character, with Marfanoid features, presents abnormal postures and slows serpentine contortions.[8-10] Likewise, this novel describes the restless legs syndrome that the waiter at an inn presents; and Mr Sharp, a teacher at David's boarding school, most likely has cervical dystonia, as the author describes an abnormal position of the neck: "carrying his head to one side... as if it were too heavy".[11-13]

The famous Bengali novelist Sarat Chandra Chattopadhyay in his famous novel Bindur Chhele (Son of Bindu), one of the central character, Bindu probably had been having some kind of seizures.

The story revolves around three characters: Annapurna, her son Amulya, and Bindubashini, a woman desperate to become a mother. Madhab's wife Bindubashini comes from an affluent family and is strikingly beautiful. Bindu is childless and when she gets to take care of Amulya, her yearning to experience motherhood finds some fulfillment. Sisters-in-law Bindu and Annapurna share a bittersweet relationship. Bindu respects Annapurna and the latter reciprocates by showering a lot of affection on her. But, they have frequent rows over household chores. During some of these, Bindu threw off "fits" with convulsive limb movements and blackouts. Whether these were true epileptic seizures or psychogenic ones are difficult to say from the inadequate semiology provided by the author. Of course, in those days, in a rural setting, medical knowledge was scanty in India. One day, they have a major disagreement over Amulya's upbringing. The disagreement proves to be irreconcilable. As a result, the two families split. The after effects of this disagreement reverberate between the two estranged families for a long time.

The great Nobel laureate poet Rabindranath Tagore mentioned about "fainting spells" in a number of female characters emotional stresses in some of his short stories where also doubt remains about their true nature—fits or faints. The height of confusion is observed in the story entitled "Jibito O Mrito" meaning Life and Death. The central character in this story is Kadambini (not to be confused with Tagore's sister-in-law Kadambari) who was a young widow, was childless, and resided in the Zamindar mansion belonging to the elder brother of her late husband. Kadambini had no surviving relatives either on her paternal or maternal side. This elder brother had a young son to whom Kadambini was deeply and affectionately attached. One day during the rains, Kadambini had a sudden "death". She was unresponsive and family members could not feel her pulse. Trying to avoid the complications arising out of an unnatural death, the family members decided to complete the cremation process in the same night. Four people set out on a long walk to the nearest cremation ground but when they reached there, thunderstorm with torrential rain started and this continued for hours. The four accompaniments left the cremation ground in search of a shelter leaving the "dead" Kadambini alone. Some hours later, Kadambini got back her senses and although she could see the trees around, she had a strange feeling what really happened to her and where she was. She left the place and started walking aimlessly. When the four accompaniments returned, they could not find Kadambini nor her clothes: they assumed that her body must had been eaten up by some man eater animals. During her aimless wandering, Kadambini met a gentleman and requested her to show her the way to a friend's house where she received a warm welcome. What had been the cause of this lady's curious illness? It is highly unlikely to be a true epileptic seizure or a simple attack of a vasovagal syncope. Was it a nonepileptic pseudoseizure status or perhaps a nonconvulsive status epilepticus attack or a dissociated state? While all three may be possible, the first one seemed more likely.

Although Kadambini was happy at her friend's house, the friend's husband started showing some extra interest toward Kadambini and this was not liked by her friend and she sent her husband to Kadambini's brother-in-laws house and arranged for her to be shifted there. As many in the said house had the impression that Kadambini had died and cremated, seeing her in person, they assumed her to be Kadambini's ghost and many started having typical hysterical fits. Her relatives were also not kind to her except the little boy whom she loved much and was addressed by him as "Auntie". In spite of this, she went into severe depression with some psychotic features and one day committed suicide by jumping into a pond in the courtyard. Tagore ends the story with the sentence: "This time ushering in a proper death, Kadambini proved to all that she did not die earlier." What really happened to her in the first instance would remain a mystery.

But the epitome of scientific divulgation through literature was Russian novelist Fyodor Dostoevsky (1821–1881), whose depictions of his own epilepsy are revealing on many facets. The writer was well conversant with the advances in neuroscience, and, in 1863, he expressed his wish to consult with the famous neurologists Armand Trousseau (1801–1867) and Moritz H Romberg (1795–1873), in Paris and Berlin respectively. In a letter to Turgenev, he expressed his curiosity about the true origin of the disease (epilepsy): "I am going to Berlin and Paris—but for the shortest possible time—for no other reason than to consult specialists in epilepsy (Trousseau in Paris, Ramberg in Berlin). There are just no specialists in Russia, and I receive such a variety of contradictory advice from the local doctors that I have lost all faith in them".[14] Nevertheless, in the same Russia that produced the great neurophysiologist Ivan Sechenov (1829–1905), Dostoevsky had consulted with a doctor in Siberia, and had a more favorable impression of him than the one expressed in his letter. "I quite unexpectedly had an epileptic fit that scared my wife to death and filled me with sadness and depression. The doctor (a learned and competent one) told me that, notwithstanding what other doctors had previously told me, I had real epilepsy and that I could expect to suffocate during one of the fits as a result of throat spasm [...] In general, he advised me to beware of the new moon (now the full moon is approaching and I expect a fit)".[14] It was Romberg (not "Ramberg" as Dostoevsky calls him in his letter) who recorded the first statistics on factors triggering seizures in epileptic patients, including the influence of the phases of the moon.[15]

What Dostoevsky experienced can be called today as ecstatic seizures. Ecstasy may be defined as a state of heightened consciousness in which an individual has a transcendent capacity for exceptional mental clarity and intensely, positive emotional experience. Ecstasy in epilepsy may apparently be considered paradoxical but this can happen. Dostoevsky wrote *"I am penetrated by an immense happiness which cannot be experienced in normal circumstances"*.[14]

The Russian novelist's life was recreated by Belarusian neuroscientist Leonid Tsypkin (1926–1982), who accompanied Dostoevsky's third and longest journey through Europe in the company of his wife. Tsypkin described the couple's reactions to an epileptic seizure of the novelist: "He was half-sitting on the rug between Anna Grigoryevna's bed and the wall, where she had dragged him, gasping under the weight of his body, and placed a pillow under his head—and his convulsions were already coming to an end, but there was foam on his lips, and so she wiped it away—and slowly opening his eyes, he looked at her without recognition".[16]

Dostoevsky's most famous novel had been *The Idiot*, first published in Russian, serially in the journal The Russian Messenger in 1868–1869. The title is an ironic reference to the central character of the novel, Lev Nikolayevich

Myshkin, a young prince whose goodness and simplicity lead many of his acquaintances to mistakenly assume that he lacks intelligence and insight. In the character of Prince Myshkin, Dostoevsky set himself the task of depicting "the positively good and beautiful man."[17] The novel reveals the results of placing such a singular individual at the center of the conflicts, desires, passions, and egoism. Joseph Frank describes *The Idiot* as "the most personal of all Dostoevsky's major works, the book in which he embodies his most intimate, cherished, and sacred convictions."[18] It includes descriptions of some of his most intense personal ordeals, such as epilepsy and mock execution, and explores moral, spiritual, and philosophical themes consequent upon them. "His primary motivation in writing the novel was to subject his own highest ideal, that of true Christian love, to the crucible of contemporary Russian society."[18] Dostoevsky himself was of the opinion that the experiment was not entirely successful, but the novel remained his favorite among his works. In a letter to Strakhov (1828–1896) (Russian philosopher, publicist, journalist, and literary critic) he wrote: "Much in the novel was written hurriedly, much is too diffuse and did not turn out well, but some of it did turn out well. I do not stand behind the novel, but I do stand behind the idea."[14]

CONCLUDING REMARKS

Transforming medical histories into novels by great authors provides a humane perspective on disease which contributes to improved doctor–patient communications. Good literature would likely make people wiser; it surely allows us to gain a more in-depth understanding of what it is to live with a disease and its sequelae, and the patient's own impression and feelings of that disease and its management.

ACKNOWLEDGMENT

The author is indebted to Ms Jana Majumdar and Ms Anuradha Majumdar for their help in the preparation of this chapter.

REFERENCES

1. Iniesta I. The Syndrome of Don Quixote. Eur J Neurol. 2010;17:545.
2. Machado MC, Lobo Antunes J. Narrative Medicine: An Optative Course at the Faculty of Medicine of Lisbon. Acta Med Port. 2016;29(12):790-2.
3. Evans M. The nightingale silenced. UK: National Library of Wales; 2009.
4. Entralgo PL. (1998). La Historia Clínica. [online] Available from https://triacastela.com/producto/la-historia-clinica/ [Last accessed February, 2025].
5. Lanska JR, Lanska DJ. Alice in Wonderland Syndrome: somesthetic vs visual perceptual disturbance. Neurology. 2013;80(13):1262-4.
6. Barbellion WNP. The Journal of a Disappointed Man, 1920. London: Chatto & Windus; 1920. p. 305.
7. Cosnett JE. Charles Dickens and epilepsy. Epilepsia. 1994;35:903-5.
8. García-Ruiz PJ. (2009). Neurology in literature: some interesting cases. The Circunvalación del Hipocampo. [online] Available from http://www.hipocampo.org/originales/original0003.asp [Last accessed February, 2025].

9. Muci-Mendoza R. Neurology in a Dickens character. Pickwickian syndrome, hypopnea sleep apneas and intracranial hypertension. Gac Med Caracas. 2009;117:154-62.
10. Schoffer KL, O'Sullivan JD. Charles Dickens: the man, medicine, and movement disorders. J Clin Neurosci. 2006;13:898-901.
11. Wainapel SF. Dickens and disability. Disabil Rehabil. 1996;18:629-32.
12. Cosnett JE. Dickens, dystonia and dyskinesia. J Neurol Neurosurg Psychiatry. 1991;54:184-7.
13. García-Ruiz PJ, Gulliksen L. Abnormal movements in David Copperfield. Neurology. 1999;14:359-6.
14. Dostoyevski FM, Frank JI, Goldstein DI. Selected letters of Fyodor Dostoevsky. New Jersey: Rutgers University Press; 1987.
15. Romberg MH. A manual of the nervous diseases of man. London: Sydenham Society; 1853.
16. Tsypkin L. Verano en Baden-Baden. Spain: Seix Barral; 2005.
17. Quintero PI. El Herbolario. Premio de Poesía Gavellar 1980. Reeditado en el poemario Almazara. Jaén: Ed Reca; 1999.
18. Iniesta I. Neurología y Literatura. Neurología. 2010;25:507-14.

CHAPTER 13

Neurology in Films

INTRODUCTION

Cinema has been defined in several different manners, but most people would agree that it should be considered both a technology and an art. Although films often depict fantasies, in many situations they also reflect real-life issues. From its earliest days, cinema got attracted to the world of health and sickness, and frequently addressed topics such as medical practice, how patients lived with their illnesses, medical ethical issues, the doctor–patient relationships, and medical research including unethical ones. The invention of film technologies in France at the end of the 19th century inspired neurologists and associated professionals to engage with this new medium to demonstrate their views on the functions of the brain, the nervous system, and the mind. Beginning with the origin of cinema in Paris, film technologies were used at La Salpêtrière, and beyond, to visualize internal mental processes, and to support the burgeoning sciences of the mind. This film-making became increasingly sophisticated by the late 1910s and early 1920s, creating innovative ways to present psychological experiences on film. Films produced by Albert Londe, Vincenzo Neri, Gheorghe Marinescu, and Jean Comandon, supported by such personalities like Charcot and Freud, were used as teaching tools for students and record interesting case studies like Charcot's hysterical seizures and gait and other movement disorders. Albert Londe and others created new filming techniques that built complexity into the visual portrayal of psychological concepts including that of "Self".[1]

Between the late 1960s and early 1980s, Frederick Wiseman filmed hundreds of hours in an emergency department, intensive care unit, and asylum.[2] These films recorded events as they happened without rehearsal and narration. Cinema and Medicine met each other in feature fiction film and in documentary format. Showing films in hospitals was revealing for both the lay audience and the medical establishment. Although they offer a narrow view of medical institutions and the issue of informed consent later became problematic, the films provide an intriguing glimpse of US healthcare and decision making. These films could have provided an invaluable resource in medical ethics in urgent care and end-of-life decision making. In more modern times, intelligent producers and film directors produced fictional films with help of professional actors to highlight mostly the social problems associated with some neurological and neuropsychiatric disorders to increase public awareness about these disorders as also to abolish or lessen social taboos associated with such disorders. Some such Western and Indian films would be briefly reviewed in this chapter.

EPILEPSY

Seizures were depicted in 20 films. Generally, seizures are used in film to develop narrative or enrich character. They serve four functions: (1) a principal character has epilepsy; thus the condition is critical to character and narrative; (2) a seizure is used to drive the narrative; (3) a seizure is used to enrich a minor role; and (4) a seizure is feigned to distract attention from another activity.[3]

Puppet Children

In the case of Angelman syndrome, a neurogenetic condition is characterized by developmental delay, absence of speech, motor impairment, happy demeanor, and seizures.[4,5] Doctor Harry Angelman himself explained the importance of his encounter with Giovanni Francesco Caroto's painting "Fanciullo con pupazzo": The boy's laughing face and the fact that his patients exhibited jerky movements gave him the idea of writing an article about the three children with a title of Puppet Children. Walt Disney presented an original depiction of it in his first full-length animated film, which displayed myoclonic jerks and a generalized tonic-clonic seizure. Like most patients with Angelman syndrome, Dopey has no speech but shows eagerness to communicate. In contrast to the absence of words, his understanding of speech is rather good, and he manages to express himself by efficient mimic and gesture. He has a wide smiling mouth and a tendency to protrude his tongue **(Fig. 1)**. His nose and chin are prominent. He

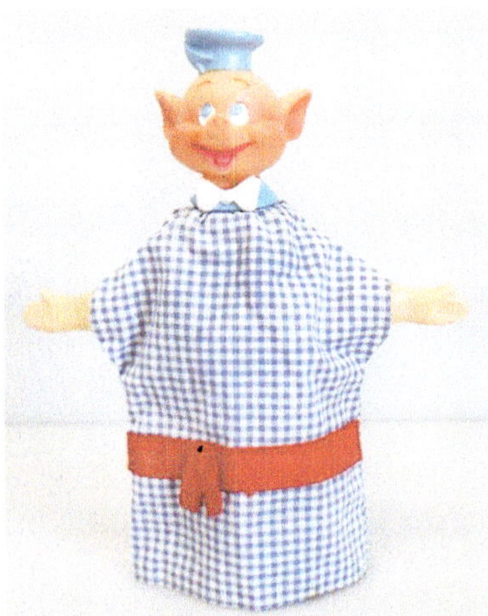

FIG. 1: "Tobey" (Angelman syndrome).

has intermittent strabismus. He has a happy disposition, enjoys playing jokes and tricks, and he can be overwhelmingly affectionate. He tends to flap his ears when he is content, as an unusual variant to the hand flapping classically seen in Angelman syndrome.[4] He has a peculiar wide-based, hopping gait, and he tends to keep his elbows flexed when he walks. He is the only one of the three with blue eyes and his head is smaller. Moreover, when it comes to washing hands, he finds himself completely immersed in the basin—a common phenomenon in this disorder.

Two Sisters (2010)

A full-length feature film on epilepsy penned and directed by Dr Debashish Chowdhury, Professor of Neurology, GB Pant Hospital, New Delhi, has won "Highly Commended Award" in an International film competition for films made on the theme of *Epilepsy* organized by ILAE (International League Against Epilepsy). The film called Two Sisters aims to sensitize people on the myths of an age-old disease which is still considered a social stigma. The film boasts of a cast that includes Soumitra Chatterjee (National Best Actor Award, 2008) and Sabyasachi Chakraborty (of Satyajit Ray's Feluda fame).

The story revolves around the family of a sociologist Dr Ashok Ganguly, his wife Alo and two daughters, Moni and Urmi **(Fig. 2)**. Moni is rejected by her fiancée's family when they come to know that she is an epileptic patient. The film marvelously captures the subtle nuances in the relationships among the family members before and after the diagnosis of this unforeseen illness. Will this family be able to gather courage to face this "stigmatized illness" and be able to seek the happiness that we all aspire? In a climactic last scene, the film probes this question and takes the audience into a plane of profound sublimity and thus is able to touch and move them deeply. It is a must watch for both doctors and lay public. The film tries to spread awareness among the masses and allay the myths

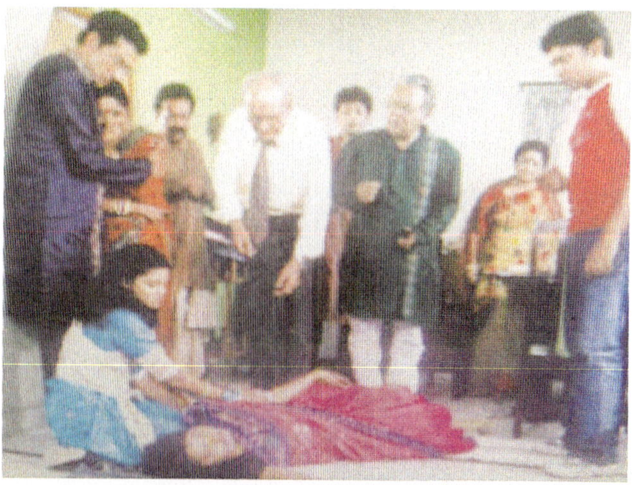

FIG. 2: A scene from Two Sisters.

and fear that surround epilepsy. It tries to bring home the message that epilepsy is a brain disease (and not a mental disease) and it can be effectively treated.

ALZHEIMER'S DISEASE

Still Alice (2014)

The lead character Dr Alice Howard is a renowned linguistics professor at Columbia University, a mother, and a wife. She started losing her speech and memory and eventually she must confront a stark reality, the diagnosis of early onset Alzheimer's disease (logopenic type) **(Fig. 3)**.

Her sense of living in the world and amidst her family started finding a new definition, and to watch it unfold is to have the viewer's heart both broken and filled with empathy.

Black (2005)

This film is really about a mixed bag of neurological disabilities and portrays the intimate relationship between a dumb mute blind girl and her teacher who was initially an alcoholic and then developed advanced Alzheimer's disease. It stars Amitabh Bachchan and Rani Mukerji in lead roles with director being Sanjay Leela Bhansali **(Fig. 4)**.

Michelle lost her eyesight and hearing after recovering from an illness at the age of 2 (probably bacterial meningitis), and grows up as a violent, uncontrollable child. Her parents, Paul and Catherine, are at their wits' end trying to control her until Debraj, an elderly alcoholic teacher, enters their lives. Debraj takes it upon himself to build Michelle into someone who can express and communicate. He

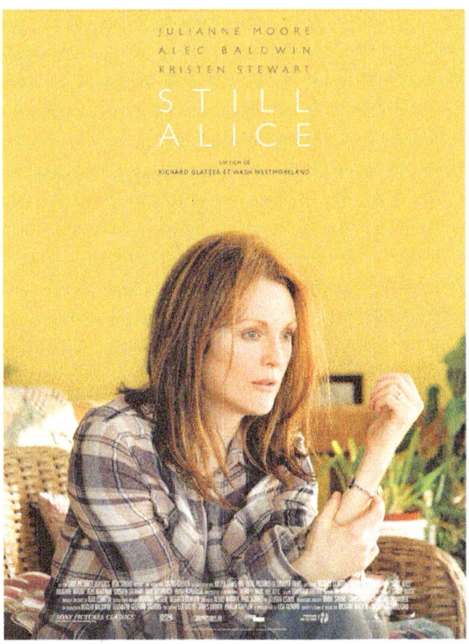

FIG. 3: A scene from Still Alice.

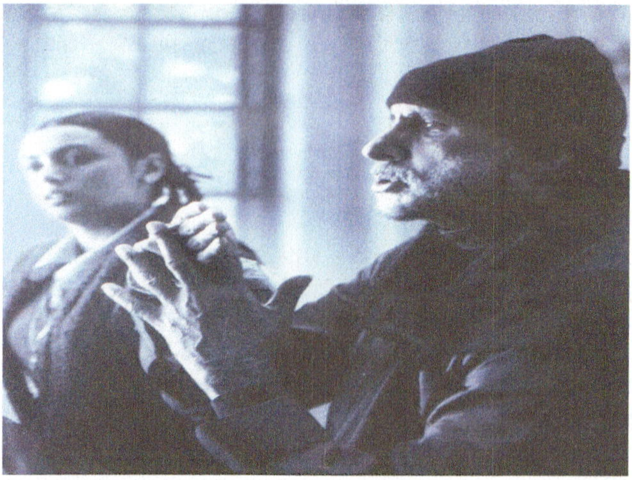

FIG. 4: A scene from Black.

uses harsh methods initially disapproved by Michelle's father, who asks him to leave. Debraj stays while her father is away on a business trip, teaching Michelle a few words and better manners. He packs his bags when Michelle's father returns. Right before he leaves, Debraj gets frustrated seeing Michelle back to being violent. He throws her into a fountain of water. It causes her to take to Debraj's lessons; she finally understands what water is, and can recognize her parents and vocalize the first syllables of small words. Debraj stays on.

Many years later, Michelle has grown into an expressive woman who is even able to dance and expertly sing. She gets admission to pursue a bachelor's degree with Debraj's help, moving away from home and living with Debraj and one of her maids. Over the next 2 years, she struggles to gain her degree, but maintains her spirit. One reason is that she must rely on Debraj for interpretation of the material but the principal helps by preparing the 1st-year course of study in *braille*. Debraj begins to succumb to *Alzheimer's disease*, at one point forgetting Michelle and leaving her stranded during a celebration. Debraj decides to leave her.

Twelve years later, Michelle manages to gain her degree and, with her proud parents looking on, gives a speech at graduation. She does not wear her ceremonial robe, insisting she would like Debraj to be the first one to see her in it. Debraj is now in a mental hospital due to his amnesia and loss of speech. Michelle visits him with her robe on; this causes flashes of memory to return as Debraj realizes she has graduated. As the window opens, Michelle reaches out to it with Debraj's hand in hers in the falling rain, and the pair say the first syllable of "water", much like the first time Michelle understood the meaning of words when Debraj threw her into the fountain. The film ends with touching scene of Michelle along with a crowd of people dressed in black carrying candles on way to a church. Amitabh left a lasting memory in the minds of all viewers and so also does young Rani Mukerji. The scene of their first experience of hesitant kissing each other is unforgettable.

STROKE

The Diving Bell and the Butterfly (2007)

Based on the true story of Elle editor, Jean-Dominique Bauby, this biographical film depicts Bauby's life after a massive stroke; a stroke which renders him almost completely paralyzed, sparing his left eye. With the help of a speech therapist, they develop a communication system in which he spells out words by blinking. Using this system, he sets himself the painstaking task of writing a memoir, a memoir which became his legacy **(Fig. 5)**.

PSYCHOLOGICAL DISORDERS

Inside Out (2015)

Made in consultation with numerous accredited psychologists, Pixar's "Inside Out" uses the vehicle of animation and children's storytelling to convey how human emotions affect interpersonal relationships. It tells the story of 11-year-old Riley who must leave behind her life in Minnesota to move to San Francisco with her family. She and her five fundamental emotions, fear, disgust, sadness, joy, and anger, must now work together to accept her new life **(Fig. 6)**.

PAROMITAR EK DIN (2000)

The Bengali (also English called The House of Memories) film explores the dual themes of friendship and loneliness; additionally, some glimpes on psycho-social issues have been addressed to **(Fig. 7)**. It starts at Sanaka's funeral where her former daughter-in-law Paromita is invited too. Paromita goes into a

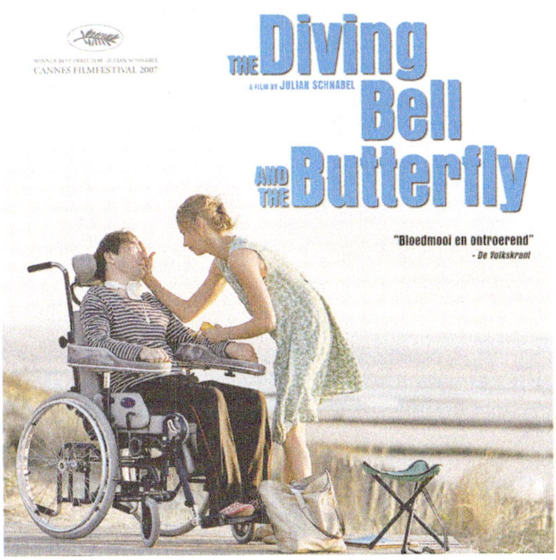

FIG. 5: A scene from The Diving Bell and The Butterfly.

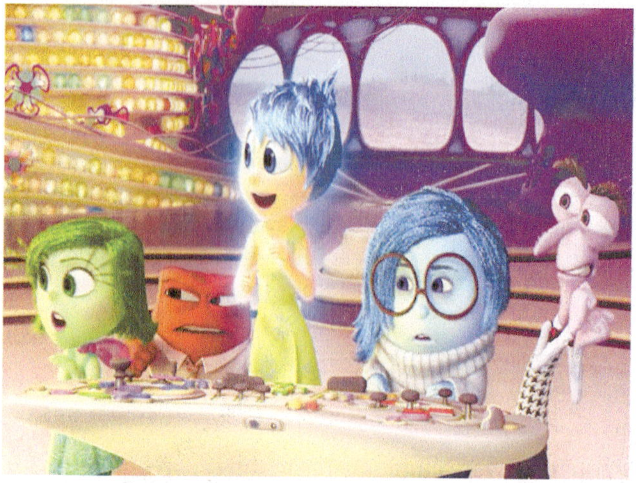

FIG. 6: A scene from Inside Out.

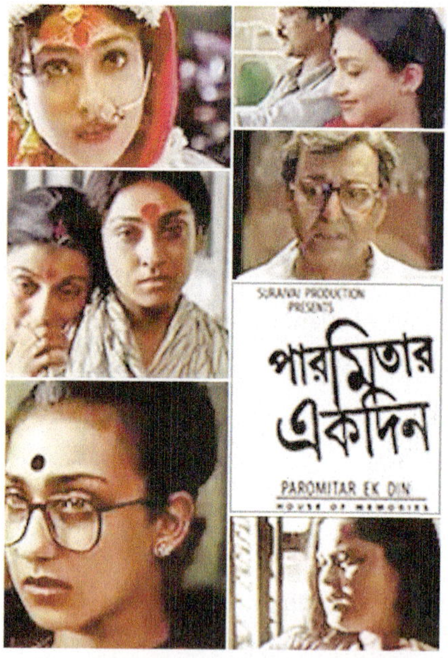

FIG. 7: Snippets from Paromitar Ek Din.

flashback where it is shown that she was previously married to Sanaka's younger son, Biru. The mother-in-law and daughter-in-law duo, Sanaka (*Aparna Sen*) and Paromita (*Rituparna Sengupta*), despite differences in age, backgrounds, and temperaments, built a strong relationship bond together. But when Paromita's marriage to Biru breaks down, social barriers prevented the women from remaining close friends. While Paromita marries Rajeev Shrivastav and begins a new life, her mother-in-law, Sanaka, is left heartbroken and alone and eventually falls seriously ill. When Paromita learns of her friend's deterioration, she is compelled to flout convention, and returned to nurse Sanaka on her deathbed; the older woman's face lighted up for a moment, registering recognition. Sanaka died a painful death of heartbreak and loneliness, leaving her family shattered. The flashback ended with Paromita leaving the funeral and discovered that she and Rajeev were expecting their first child.

What were the bonds that bind Sanaka and Paromita together? Apart from the fact that they were two women married into the same family, to father and son, there were two elements they had in common. One, both of them were not happy in their marriages. Two, Sanaka had a daughter who had schizophrenia and Paromita's little boy was a spastic child. And here comes the socio-neuropsychiatric aspect of the film. Sanaka's 27-year-old daughter (Khuku) is portrayed as a schizophrenic. However, from the nature of her behavior, it seemed more likely an Attention Deficit Hyperactivity Disorder with some element of Impulse Control Disorder. She could sing beautifully, play the tune in her tanpura, took care of her mother's medicines after Paromita left the house, and even tried to take care of Paromita's first child and feed the pigeons. On the social side, the girl Khuku was mishandled and even beaten by both Sanaka and her sons. This highlights the sad life of mentally and psychologically challenged people in the family and society. Somewhat similar fate awaited the little spastic child born to Paromita and Biru and this was not only looked down upon and commented on by other members of the family, it was the major reason for separation between Paromita and Biru (who blamed each other's family for this ill-fated incident). There is a scene where the mother and daughter-in-law are shown soaping each other. Some critics have said that there is a possible lesbian shade in the love between Sanaka and Paromita. But, this is incorrect. In extended Bengali families, women bathing and soaping each other was not uncommon. To sum up, *Paromitar Ek Din* is a culture-specific Bengali film which reflects the transgenerational suppressed aggression in women within the much talked about joint family structure, exploding right into the politically correct face of the Bengali bhadralok.

AUTISM SPECTRUM DISORDER

My Name is Khan (2007)

An Indian Muslim man with Asperger's syndrome (one form of autism spectrum disorder where affected persons tend to have a hard time relating to others socially; they usually stick to a very specific routine, have a narrow set of interests, and act in repetitive ways such as flapping their hands), played by the famous actor Shah Rukh Khan, takes a challenge to speak to the President of the United States seriously and embarks on a cross-country journey **(Fig. 8)**. During November 2007, San Francisco-based autistic Rizwan Khan, en route to meet the President of the USA so that he can convey that his name is Khan and he is not a terrorist, recalls his life, initially with his Bombay-based dad, Dilawar Amanaullah Khan; mom, Razia; and brother, Zakir. Dilawar works for the State Transport workshop in Borivali, and Rizwan accompanies him, learns the trade, and can repair virtually anything. After his passing, Rizwan is abused

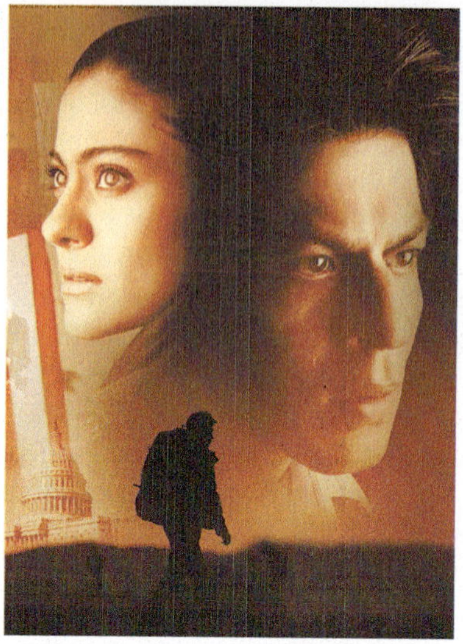

FIG. 8: A scene from My Name is Khan.

by his classmates, as well as by Zakir, who feels neglected, so she hires Wadia to teach Rizwan. Years later, Zakir decides to relocate to USA, and, once there, gets married to Hasina. He sponsors Razia and Rizwan, but Razia passes away. In San Francisco, where Zakir runs "Mehnaz Herbal Beauty Products", Rizwan is hired as a door-to-door salesman, while Hasina concludes that he has Asperger's syndrome. While selling products, he meets with and is attracted to a Hindu Salon worker, Mandira Rathod, a single mother of Sameer, whose husband abandoned her and relocated to Australia. Both Rizwan and Mandira decide to get married much to Zakir's chagrin, who asks Rizwan to leave. The trio relocate to Banville, open their own salon, encounter racial profiling after the 9-11 terrorist attacks, are blacklisted, shunned and suffer losses, and then Sameer gets killed. Mandira blames Rizwan for her plight, while she decides to pursue Sameer's death with Detective Miguel Garcia. When tragedy strikes, Mandira is devastated and they split. Rizwan is confused and very upset that the love of his life has left him. To win her back, he embarks on a touching and inspiring journey across America.

Barfi

Murphy Johnson (Ranbir Kapoor), also known as Barfi, is an optimistic, street-wise, charming young man born deaf and mute to a lower middle-class Nepali family in Darjeeling. His mother died while giving birth to him and his father, Jungbahadur (Akash Khurana), raised him as a single parent while working as a chauffeur. Barfi is known to be a troublemaker—he cuts lamp posts, plays practical jokes on innocent people, and is often pursued comically by Inspector Sudhanshu Dutta (Saurabh Shukla), a local police officer. Barfi meets Shruti Ghosh (Ileana D'Cruz), a gorgeous, educated young girl, who is new in Darjeeling. She is engaged to a rich man, Ranjeet Sengupta (Jisshu Sengupta), and is due to get married in 3 months. Barfi is smitten by her heavenly beauty and tries to woo her. Shruti also falls in love with Barfi, but her mother (Roopa Ganguly) dissuades her from pursuing him, pointing out that he could not take care of her with his disabilities and lack of money. Shruti unwillingly agrees to her mother's advice, gets married to Ranjeet, and leaves the town, breaking all contact with Barfi.

Shortly after Shruti's departure, Jungbahadur loses his job as a chauffeur and suffers from kidney failure, compelling Barfi to somehow raise ₹7,000 for his hospital treatment. After an unsuccessful attempt of robbing a local bank due to Inspector Dutta's intervention, Barfi contemplates the kidnapping of Jhilmil Chatterjee (Priyanka Chopra), his autistic childhood friend and wealthy heiress of her late grandfather's fortune, for a ransom. Upon arriving, Barfi finds out that she has already been kidnapped from her house and spots her in an unattended van. He sneaks in and drives Jhilmil away from the ransom delivery. Barfi proceeds to hide her in his apartment with the police in pursuit and delivers a ransom note pasted with words in newspaper cut-outs to Jhilmil's wealthy father, Durjoy Chatterjee (Ashish Vidyarthi). Although Barfi is able to collect the ransom from Jhilmil's father, he is aghast to discover that Jungbahadur has died just as he makes the hospital payment. Dejected, Barfi tries to leave Jhilmil at her caretaker's village, but she refuses to leave him and the two soon move to Kolkata, where Barfi assumes responsibility for Jhilmil and strives hard to take care of her.

Six years later, Barfi and Shruti reunite by fate in a street-side utensil shop. Shruti is unhappy with her marriage with Ranjeet and tries to rekindle her friendship with Barfi, much to chagrin of the lovestruck Jhilmil, who then goes missing in the city. Shruti files a missing complaint for Jhilmil and Inspector Dutta influenced the Darjeeling police to resume their pursuit of Barfi and arrest him. During the process of interrogation, another ransom demand for Jhilmil is made and she is apparently killed in the process of exchange, though her dead body is never discovered. In order to conclude the case, the police decide to frame Barfi for Jhilmil's murder. Inspector Dutta, who grew fond of Barfi after pursuing him for his nuisances, asks Shruti to take him away, offering him a second chance in life. Shruti agrees and hopes that since now Jhilmil is gone, she can finally be with Barfi.

However, Barfi is deeply affected by Jhilmil's loss and finds living with Shruti unfulfilling. Eventually, he stumbles upon Jhilmil's special-care home address on the scribbles that she had made in their house. Barfi takes Shruti to the location to search for her and the two learn that Jhilmil has been alive all along, and that both the kidnappings were fabricated by her father so that he could embezzle money from Jhilmil's trust fund. In the second attempt, the second time, Jhilmil's father and the special-care home owner, Daju (Haradhan Bandopadhyay), together faked her death, so that Jhilmil could return to her special-care home, away from her alcoholic mother (Preeti Mamgain). Barfi and Jhilmil have a happy reunion at the special-care home and the two are married, while Shruti spends the rest of her days alone, prosperous, having lost her chance to be with Barfi.

Several years later, an elderly Barfi is shown to be seriously ill and on his deathbed at the hospital. Jhilmil lies with him on the hospital bed, while Shruti narrates how they both died peacefully, not wanting to leave each other behind in life or death. The film ends with the happy days of Barfi and Jhilmil in their old age at the special-care home and the credits roll **(Fig. 9)** (adapted from *www.wikipedia.com*).

Rain Man (1988)

Car dealer, Charlie Babbitt, learns that his father has died and returns home to discover that he has an older autistic brother who lives in a mental facility, and that the facility has been left their father's $3 million fortune. With money in his eyes, he checks his brother out of the facility and together they embark on a cross-country journey back to Los Angeles in which the beauty of brotherhood is unmasked **(Fig. 10)**.

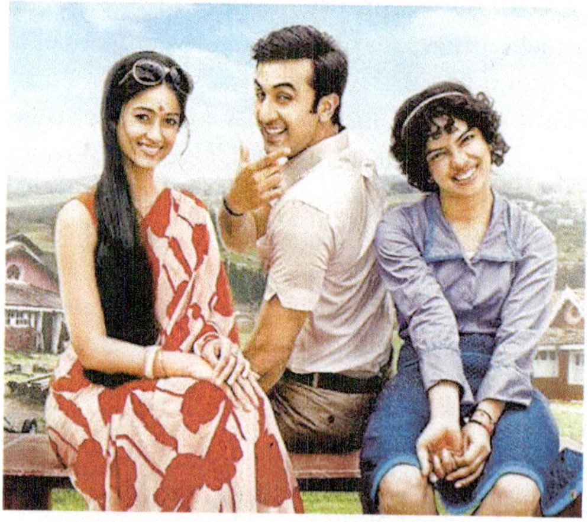

FIG. 9: A scene from Barfi.

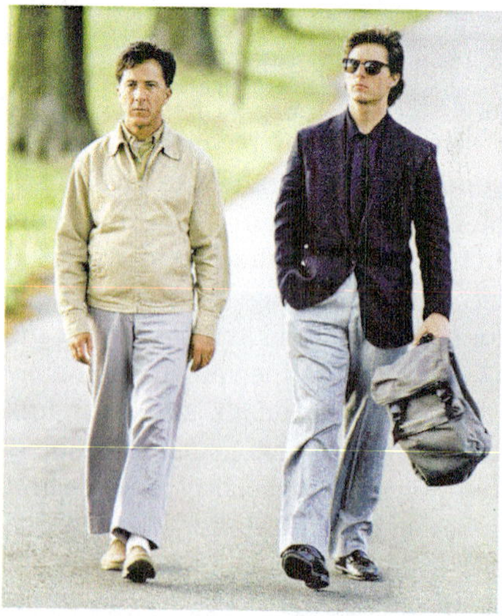

FIG. 10: A scene from Rain Man.

DYSLEXIA

Taare Zameen Par (2007)

The film *Taare Zameen Par* (Stars upon the Ground), a Hindi movie released toward the end of 2007, was a big box-office hit **(Fig. 11)**. The script was written by Amole Gupta and Deepa Bhatia and the film was directed by the noted actor Aamir Khan. The film portrays the life of a young boy, Ishaan Awasthi (enacted by 8-year-old Darsheel Safary), who is dyslexic and cannot read or write; he leads a tormented life until he meets with his art teacher, Ramashankar Nikumbh (enacted by Amir Khan), who discovers his artistic talents. In the film,[6] *Taare Zameen Par*, the child Ishaan Awasthi is ridiculed at school and at home for not being able to write and read properly. He has developmental dyslexia.

He seems to be of average intelligence and his spontaneous speech is fluent and meaningful. From the very beginning of the film, his facial expression appears very innocent, but it is tinged with stupidity. In fact, though he is "stupid," he has the intelligence to get his letter requesting absence from school written by his elder brother. Ishaan cannot read, and his writing contains several spelling mistakes and the use of inappropriate letters and words.

He is frustrated and this is evident through his behavior at times (kicking flower pots) but he has no other conduct disorder. His apparent hyperactivity (shown in a scene of his taking a shower) is perhaps a normal phenomenon in children of his age. However, he certainly lacks motor skills (as is known to occur in dyslexia) as he cannot knot his tie or tie his shoelaces properly. His inability to perform simple arithmetic is a bit of a puzzle; this is unusual in dyslexia. Ishaan does not have dyscalculia, he has a prominent language deficit. Perhaps, this has been portrayed to enhance the image of helplessness and disability in this young boy. At times, the boy looks vacant, absorbed in his own thoughts. Such behaviors (daydreaming, perhaps) are not unusual in his age and such cases are often referred to neurologists as possible absence seizure spells. The film has a

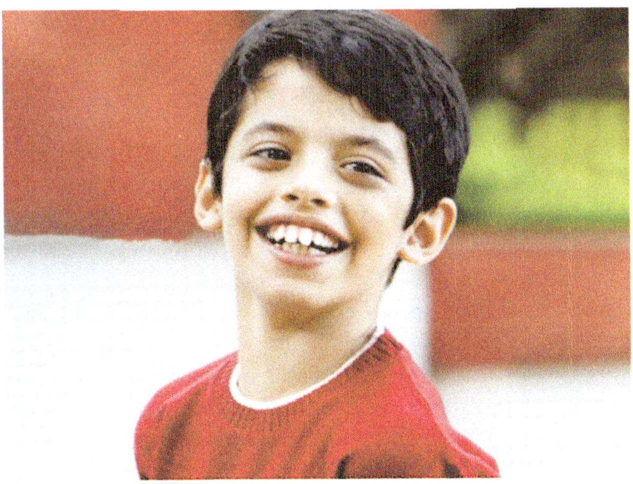

FIG. 11: Darsheel as Ishaan, the dyslexic child in the film.

happy ending, however, with Ishaan's artistic talent being discovered by his art teacher Ramashankar Nikumbh. In fact, his art teacher makes the diagnosis of dyslexia after examining Ishaan's class notebooks. The discovery of Ishaan's artistic talent and the way it blooms under the care of his art teacher is the most important (and joyous) neurocognitive phenomenon in the film. Ishaan's case seems to be related to the phenomenon of "disinhibition" of his right parietal lobe (Ishaan is right-handed and hence his right parietal lobe must be the nondominant one) which is related in turn to the developmental delay of his left hemisphere (the dominant hemisphere) that is manifested in his developmental dyslexia. Ishaan Awasthi may thus be labeled as an example of "dyslexic savant syndrome." Furthermore, the improvement in his artistic skill triggered by the support of his art teacher (Ishaan went on to receive the first prize in the school painting competition) highlights a major and therapeutically important issue in cognitive neuroscience and neuropsychology—namely cosmetic neurology.

Dyslexic characters have featured in a number of works of fiction. Notable works include Henry Winkler's Hank Zipper series of children's books and Jennifer Weiner's novel "In Her Shoes," which was adapted as a film in 2005. Taki Wartooth and Skwisgaar Skwigelf both from the TV show "Metalocalypse" claim to be dyslexic, as they cannot read music. "Shooting Fish" features Dylan, a dyslexic conman, who makes his living using confidence tricks to gain money from rich people. He justifies his lifestyle by claiming that he is unable to get a job because of his dyslexia. Additionally, there are three episodes of the "The Cosby Show" which focus on dyslexia, all three having Theo as one of the major characters in the plot. George Lopez from the eponymous TV show has dyslexia (*source*: https://www.wikipedia.com).

In remedial training in children with dyslexia, it is important to facilitate the development of their unique artistic and other abilities to its full capacity rather than to overemphasize on the correction of the disturbed coded symbol operations. This film should be an eyeopener to parents of dyslexic children. The entire team and in particular the young artist, Darsheel, who so vividly portrays the helplessness of a disabled child, deserve our appreciation.

PORTRAYAL OF COMA IN FILMS[7]

Thirty movies from 1970 to 2004, with actors depicting prolonged coma, were reviewed by the authors (Wijdicks EFM, and Wijdicks CA). Accurate depiction of comatose patients was assessed by appearance, the intensity of care, determination of the exact cause of coma and probability of awakening, and appropriate compassionate exchanges between the medical personnel and family members. Twenty-two key scenes from 17 movies were rated for accuracy by a panel of intensivists and critical care nurses and then were shown to an audience of 72 nonmedical viewers. Accuracy of the scenes was assessed using a special scale. Coma was most often caused by motor vehicle accidents or violence (63%). The time in a comatose state varied from days to 10 years. Awakening occurred in 18 of 30 motion pictures (60%). Awakening was sudden with cognition intact, even after prolonged coma. Actors personified "Sleeping Beauty" (eyes closed, beautifully groomed). Physicians appeared as caricatures. Only two movies had a reasonable accurate representation (Dream Life of Angels and Reversal of Fortune). The majority of the surveyed viewers identified inaccuracy of representation of coma, awakenings, and conversations on the experience of being in a coma, except in 8 of the 22 scenes (36%). About 40% of the 72 nonmedical viewers could potentially allow these scenes to influence decision making in real life. It was felt by the authors that misrepresentation of coma and awakening was common in motion pictures and impacted on the public perception of coma.

WHAT HAD BEEN THE ROLE OF NEUROLOGISTS IN FILMS?

"Those damn neurologists, they think they can run the world" (EDtv, 1999). Neurologists are rarely very favorite with producers and directors. Rather, their appearance in films is often brief, with playwriters preferring surgeons, psychiatrists, and family doctors. The neurologist is often portrayed in film as a caricature character: the patient—aloof neuroscientist studying a rare neurological disease, the strictly business and cynical physician, the award hungry researcher undertaking highly unethical human experiments—are just some such examples. In the USA, the film Awakenings introduced the neurologist to cinemagoers, with Robin Williams as the fictional Dr Sayer portraying real-life Oliver Sacks. Williams played a bearded, spectacled, coy neurologist discovering a treatment for encephalitis lethargica with parkinsonian features **(Fig. 12)**.

In The Royal Tenenbaums, the neurologist Raleigh St Clair (Bill Murray) is also modeled on Oliver Sacks. In the film, Dr St Clair writes a book entitled The Peculiar Neurodegenerative Inhabitants of the Kazawa Atoll featuring amnesia, dyslexia, and color blindness combined with a highly acute sense of hearing. After a patient is subjected to a block design test revealing grossly incongruent result, the neurologist chuckles, "My goodness, how interesting, how bizarre." Shocking....is not it?

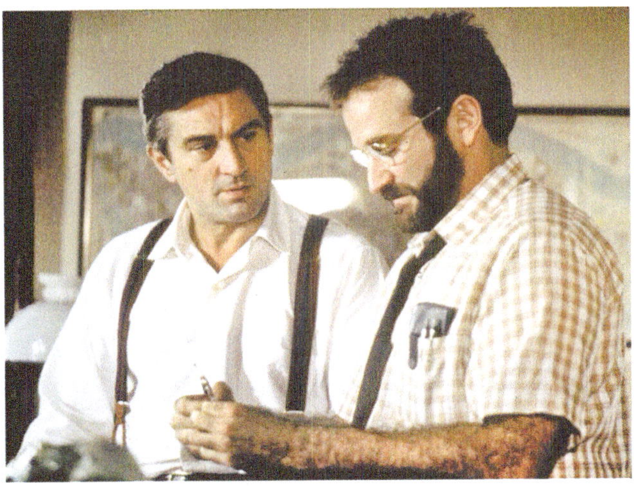

FIG. 12: A scene from Awakenings.

For the first time, a feature film—the César-nominated Augustine—is devoted fully to neurologist Jean Martin Charcot. If any neurologist seemed to have "run the world", it must have been Charcot.[8] Charcot's studies of female hysteria cemented his international fame. He was well known for his clinical demonstrations showing the effects of touching "hysterogenic zones" that would induce a hysterical attack. His treatment of young afflicted women (and also men) included hypnosis and, most memorably and shown in this movie, the "compresseur ovarien" (an abdominal vice with a knob that applied pressure to the ovary), both of which could abort the spells. In the film, Charcot is played by Vincent Lindon, but he has little of Charcot's imposing stature and manners (Napoleonic). Nonetheless, the film recreates the atmosphere at La Salpêtrière and Charcot's associates reasonably well. Some aspects of neurological examination, the major discrepancies, and rapid changes in symptomatology are shown and generally correct. The manifestations of "la grande hystérie" are exhibited by Augustine, played well by Stéphanie Sokolinski (Soko), and the audience gets quite a show, including the well-known "arc-en-circle" position of a hysterical patient **(Fig. 13)**.

While serving at a dinner party, kitchen maid Augustine feels her hands going numb and then has a violent fit that leaves her paralyzed in one eye. Augustine is brought to a hospital where she attracts the attention of Jean-Martin Charcot after she has seizures in front of him. Charcot examines her while she is naked and realizes that she has lost feeling in one side of her body. He pierces her arm with a hot needle, but Augustine cannot feel it. He also discovers that despite having matured physically, Augustine has never menstruated. He has Augustine hypnotized in front of the doctors and induces one of her fits which results in her having an orgasm before collapsing. The doctors applaud Charcot and he begins to work with Augustine in earnest, giving her own room within the hospital and examining her thoroughly. The more time they spend together, the more Charcot begins to feel attracted to Augustine, even sneaking into her room

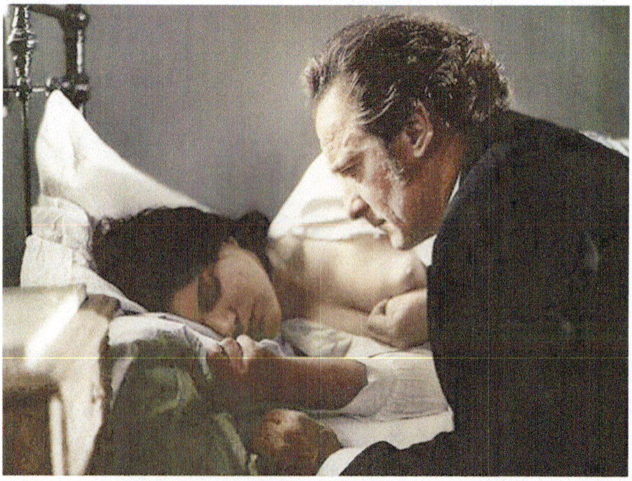

FIG. 13: A scene from Augustine (2012).

at night to observe her sleeping. Conversely, Augustine begins to feel trapped. When her cousin stops visiting her, Augustine decides she wants to leave and find employment. Charcot refuses to let her, promising he will help her when he cures her. Charcot finally receives the go-ahead to lecture in front of the medical academy with Augustine. However, as she is being prepped to go to the lecture, she runs away, falls down a set of steps, hits her head, and regains sensation in her body. When Charcot tries to hypnotize her for his lecture in order to induce a seizure, the hypnotization fails and Augustine whispers to Charcot that she is cured, flexing her hand for him. After Charcot tells his audience that some experiments are best left to the lab, Augustine fakes an attack of hysteria.

Unfortunately, some viewers chose to label Augustine as nothing more than a psychoerotic thriller. The director's goal might have been to show a chauvinistic doctor's behavior and sexual desire evoked by lusty women—and indeed, in the culminating scene, Charcot having sex with her in his office. What a shame!! A feature film rarely provides useful insights into the practices of a neurologist or in essence of any doctor.

CONCLUDING REMARKS: NEUROLOGY IN FILMS AND NEUROCINEMA

So far in this essay we have discussed the portrayal of different neurological diseases in films through acting by experienced actors to highlight to the audience the cardinal features of individual diseases, the mode and extent of their suffering, the ways the patients (actors) adopted to cope with their disabilities, the reactions of the family and the society at large to the diseased state, and, at times, the strategies adopted by the affected subjects or their caregiver to rise above the situation. All these had been done by the producers or directors of the films to increase public awareness about the disease, remove social taboos about the disease, and thus make life more tolerable for the sufferers of such diseases living in real-life situations. Neurocinema is a vastly different newly developed discipline to look at the brain's responses while viewing a film and the effect it leaves on the mind.[9] Cinema, which in essence is a combination of technology and art, is a multidimensional art capable of affecting the neurophysiology of our central nervous system in different ways. Studies show that different parts of the brain are activated while watching a fiction film and consequently, the movie evokes consciousness. This enables cinema to deeply influence the brain's functions. The effect and its nature are the main themes of the newly emerged science of neurocinema. Perhaps, one of the most striking qualities of a movie is its flow. We are facing a series of events which are frequently and connectively targeting our minds like daily issues but with a purposeful and relevant content. Is it possible then to say that filmmaking process rebuilds the contents of consciousness. Consciousness does not refer to the activity of a certain area of the brain or a specific type of neurons; instead, it is the result of a dynamic, flowing relationship between a vast range of neurons. The thalamocortical system is a major structure for conscious activity. The system is not only internally connected but is also linked to other parts of the brain. On the other hand, the content of our consciousness is associated with different parts of the cortex. Neurophysiologically, this complex system forms our consciousness power. Hasson et al.[10] examined the brain response and activity while watching a movie. He used fMRI in this study as well as a new method called "inter-subject correlation (ISC) analysis." Using this method, the degree of similarity in brain activities of different viewers could be measured, which plays an important role in neurocinematic study because important aspects of studying brain responses to a movie are not equal, and reactions of a considerable number of viewers need to be investigated to study the pattern of brain activation. Such studies would be of interest in filmography and for professional film critics. Why are the opinions of critics about fictional movies similar or dissimilar? Why are viewers sometimes get fascinated by a particular movie? Why are some scenes memorable? Some clues to these questions may be found through results of fMRI and ISC studies done on a large number of viewers and film critics. Neurocinema as a multidisciplinary science can help us to study the relationship between movies and minds.

REFERENCES

1. Evans B. The origins of film, psychology and the neurosciences. Hist Human Sci. 2024;37(2): 12-40.
2. Wijdicks EFM. Teaching medicine through film: Wiseman's medical trilogy revisited. BMC Med Educ. 2019;19(1):387.
3. Kerson JF, Kerson TS, Kerson LA. The Depiction of Seizures in Film. Epilepsia. 1999;40(8): 1163-7.
4. Angelman H. 'Puppet' Children: A report on three cases. Dev Med Child Neurol. 1965;7: 681-8.
5. Dan B, Christiaens F. Dopey's seizure. Seizure. 1999;8:238-40.
6. Chakravarty A. Taare Zameen Par and dyslexic savants. Ann Indian Acad Neurol. 2009;12: 99-103.
7. Wijdicks EFM, Wijdicks CA. The portrayal of coma in contemporary motion pictures. Neurology. 2006;66(9):1300-3.
8. St-Denis A, Massie R. Charcot and recent French cinema. J Hist Neurosci. 2024:1-10. Online ahead of print.
9. Naser Moghadasi A. Neurocinema: A brief overview. Iran J Neurol. 2015;14(3):180-4.
10. Hasson U, Landesman O, Knappmeyer B, Vallines I, Rubin N, Heeger DJ. Neurocinematics: The Neuroscience of Film. Projections. 2008;2(1):1-26.

CHAPTER 14

Ardhanarishvara: A Study in Religious Philosophy, Scientific Mysticism, and Neuroscience

INTRODUCTION

In Hinduism, Ardhanarishvara or Ardhanari is an androgynous deity composed of Shiva and his consort Shakti (Parvati), representing the synthesis of masculine and feminine forces. The term is derived from union of three words—Ardha (half), Nari (female), and Ishvara (God or Goddess). The Ardhanari form also illustrates how the female principle of God is inseparable from the male principle of God, Shiva. Ardhanari in iconography is depicted as half-male and half-female, split down the middle. The best sculptural depictions of Shiva as Ardhanari are found in the sensuous Chola dynasty (900–1300 AD) bronzes in Southern India and the sculptures of Ellora (near Aurangabad in India) and Elephanta (near Mumbai). The earliest Ardhanarishvara images are reported from the early period of Kushanas (c 35–60 AD). The early Kushana rulers were, however, not Hindus; they were probably Buddhists and Western culture had a great influence on their artworks. A sculpture depicting only the head of Ardhanarishvara is preserved at the Mathura museum, Mathura, India dating to about 500 AD probably belonging to the time of Gupta dynasty who were Hindus.[1]

ICONOGRAPHY (FIG. 1)

Barring a few exceptions, the left halves or the Ardhanari sculptures comprise male anatomy and the right halves (viewer's left and right), that of the female. However, a reverse disposition has also been noted probably created by sculptures belonging to the Shakti sect (devotees of Shakti). In both sculptures and paintings, the feminine characters are more obvious (more so in the paintings) and I shall make a comment about this later in the article.

The female part, in general, imparts a feeling of elegance and tenderness especially because of the elegantly curved prominent breast. The image may be endowed with two, three, four, six, and eight arms. Imagination and depiction of multiple body parts are often essential features in Hindu conception of gods and goddesses and even demons. Durga in Eastern India is often sculptured

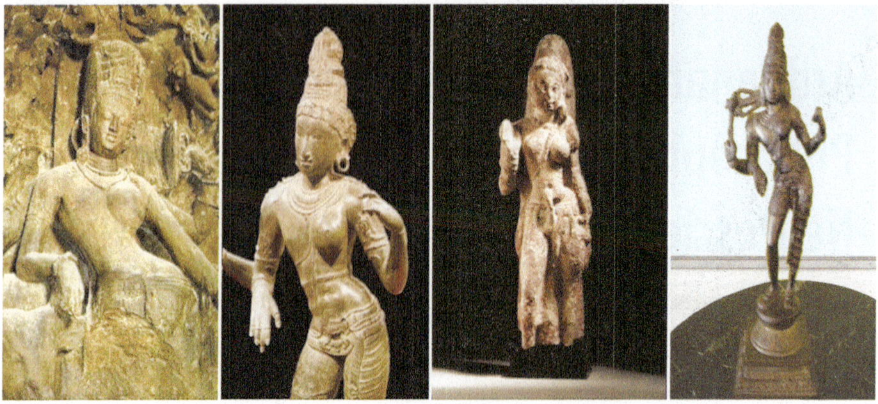

FIG. 1: Ardhanarishvara: Iconography. The first sculpture on the left is at Elephanta and the last one on the right is a small replica of the Chola bronze.

with ten hands and Ravana, the demon King, with as many heads. In Ardhanari, arms more than eight are attribute of Rudra Shiva who has been conceived with as many as thousand arms. The two-armed image is the Ardhanarishvara, in *lalita* posture, the beautiful one in absolute ease. The female hand carries either a mirror or a *nilotpala*, a blue lotus. The male hand either rests on the bull (often identified with sculptures of Shiva and called Nandi) or is let loose below the thigh. It may also be in *abhaya mudra*, the gesture of imparting fearlessness or giving blessings. When three armed, one is generally on the female side and two on the male side. Of the two, one is often in *abhaya* or *varada mudra* and the other one carries a trident (Trishula—the divine weapon of Shiva). In four-armed figures, the two male hands are generally the same as above, but the second female hand may carry either a mirror or *nilotpala* or a pot. In the six- and eight-armed figures, the extra male hands carry various weapons like a small hand-held drum (Damaru) and the additional female arms may carry a parrot in addition to mirror, lotus, or pot **(Fig. 2)**.

Overall, the images have three body postures—the *abhanga*, a posture without a curve, the *tribhanga*, a posture with three body curves, and the *atibhanga*, a posture with extreme curves. The body curves give elegance to the images and such curves are commonly observed in many ancient Indian art forms and give a feeling of dynamism to the image increasing its aesthetic value.[2,3] Recent sculptors have, at times, conceived of this dual image in the sitting posture as well, but this is not common. It is of interest to note that at Elephanta, there exists also a three-faced image (sculpture) of Shiva Maheshwara—on the left, his male profile displaying virility and willpower, on the right his female aspect (viewer's side) gentle charming and seductive—and in the center the sublime union of the two aspects in the magnificent head.

The present author has, in his collection, an antique bronze sculpture which cannot strictly be called Ardhanari but depicts the union of Goddess Kali (Shakti) and Shiva in one rounded piece **(Fig. 3)**. Here, the protruding tongue represents the Goddess Kali and the moustache, the sickle-shaped moon and the Trishula

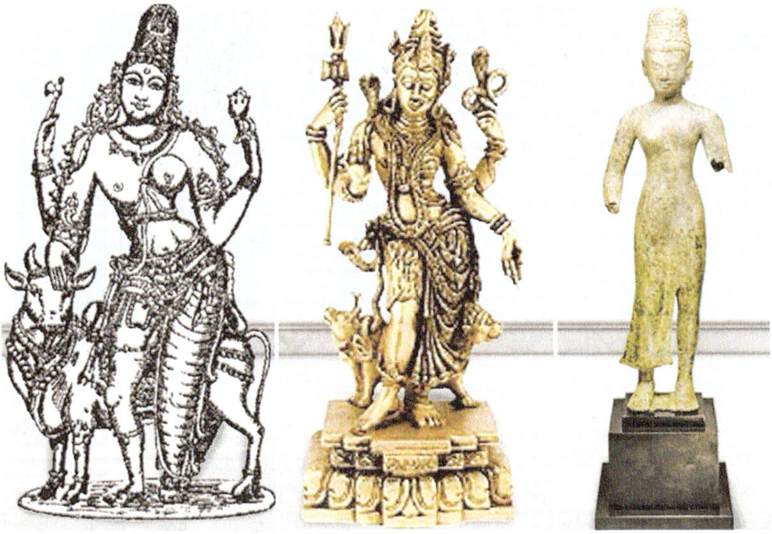

FIG. 2: Ardhanarishvara variability: The first two sculptures from the left display multiple limbs while the third one, from Cambodia, the left half of the sculpture is female—the reverse of the one commonly encountered.

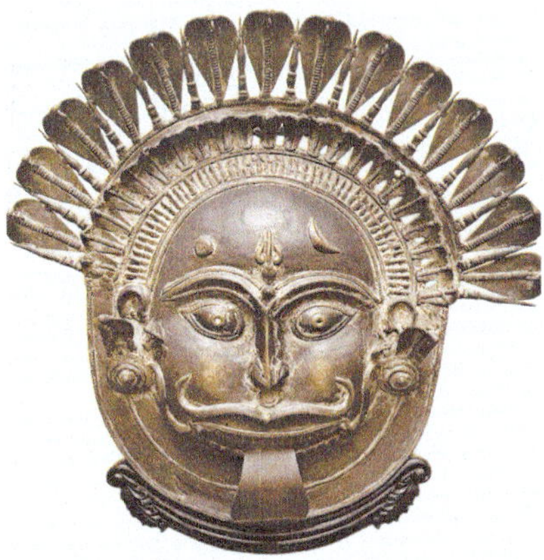

FIG. 3: The unorthodox bronze sculpture depicting an union of Goddess Kali and Shiva.

on the forehead, and the row of snake heads around the head are components of Shiva, the male consort of Shakti or Parvati or Kali. The basic religious philosophy underlying the union of Shiva and Shakti in one piece is maintained.

RELIGIOUS PHILOSOPHY

The basic concept of combining a male God (Shiva) with a female Goddess (Shakti or Parvati) speaks of a combination of two opposing forces in one image. This conception of duality of existence suggests "Dvaita" which contradicts the fundamental concept of God in the Advaita Veda. In the Shaiva philosophy of Advaitabad, God is single who also is the cause of the entire existence and it is by his will and act of him that the cosmos came into being. However, in the Shaivite hymn (of followers of Shiva), "*Ekohum bahusyam*" (Shiva Purana), i.e., I am one, but wishes to be many, there echoes the Rig Vedic perception of the single egg splitting into *bhuta* (soul) and *prana* (life). This apart, most interpretations of the Vedas widely favor the principle of monogenic existence. Besides its emphasis on the unity of the outward duality, the Rig Veda acclaims that the male is only so much male as much he is female and vice-versa the female is only as much female as much she is male. The maleness and femaleness are attributes contained in one frame. The *Smarta* tradition, which, by and large, follows Advaita philosophy, believes all forms, male and female, to be different forms of the impersonal absolute, Brahman, who is of neuter gender and can never be defined. Brahman is viewed as without personal attributes (Nirguna Brahman) or with attributes (Saguna Brahman) as God. In Advaita Vedanta, Ishvara (generally meaning Saguna Brahman) is simply the manifest form of Brahman upon the human mind. Thus, according to Smarta views, the divine can be with attributes, Saguna Brahman, and can be viewed with whatever attributes (a male god or a female goddess) a devotee conceives.[3]

Apart from Brahman, from whom the cosmos or universe originated, the other two great Gods in Hinduism are Vishnu and Shiva. With a broadened philosophical view, all three can be assumed to be the same or different forms of the same force. However, opinions vary, depending upon conception of the writers of the Vedas. In Vaishnavism and Shaivism which are exclusive monotheistic denominations of Hinduism and like Christian or Muslim tradition, God (whoever he is), Vishnu or Shiva, is personified as male when in fact God transcends gender and gender is simply used for embodied human beings to worship.[4] For example, Shaivites and Vaishnavites worship God in nonanthropometric images, the "Linga" and "Shaligram", respectively. Furthermore, the principle that God's true nature is sexless is emphasized in the Vishnu Sahasranama, a prayer reciting the one thousand names of Vishnu. The names focus not on his sex or anthropometric form but highlight his inherent nature or characters such as pervading the universe and as destroyer of sin. While to a common man, Vishnu (as well as Shiva) is commonly portrayed with human features, scholars clearly state that Vishnu (and Shiva) pervades everything and is not anthropometric. He has no particular shape or form, can manifest in any form, and is the center of all forces. He is the inducting spirit in all beings and the whole cosmos constitute his body. Like Christianity and Islam, God transcends gender but both Vishnu and Shiva have been traditionally referred to using grammatical gender. On the other hand, while God is conceived as a male, his power is often viewed in the female form of Shakti. However, God and his power are indivisible, unitary, and the same. The analogy is that fire represents God and the actual heat, the Shakti. In Ardhanari, Lord Shiva assumed a form and split into two halves of male and female—the union of substance and energy—the being and his force (Shakti). At this stage, it is important to comment on the concept of Shakti in Hinduism. Shakti is also known as Parvati, Uma, Durga, and Kali and generally considered the female consort of Shiva. Devotees of Shakti are known as Shaktas. The great scholar NN Bhattacharyya in his "History of Shakta Religion"[5] explains the basic concept of Shakti. He writes "... (they) who worship the supreme Deity as exclusively a female principle... conceive their Great Goddess as the personification of primordial energy and the source of all divine and cosmic evolution. She is identified with the Supreme Being, conceived as the source and the spring as well as the controller of all the forces and potentialities of nature. Nowhere in the religious history of the world do we come across such a completely female oriented system".[5] Here we see a conflict, while the devotees of Shiva (Shaivites) believe that Shakti is a part of Shiva, the Shaktas would look at the relation the other way round.[6] This would lead to a different interpretation of the Ardhanarishvara. In one concept, it is basically a Shiva deity with one part of it depicted as Shakti, on the other it is basically a female Goddess (Shakti) one part of which is male. The Shaivite scholars argue that the feminine manifest is ultimately only the vehicle through which the masculine unmanifest Parasiva is ultimately reached. Here, the Divine Mother (Shakti) becomes something of a mediator, who bestows *advaitic moksha* (eternal freedom or peace) on those who worship her. Thus, these Shaivite views often conclude that Shaktism is effectively a subdenomination of Shaivism, arguing that Devi (Shakti) is worshipped to attain union with Shiva, who in Shaktism is the impersonal unmanifest absolute. This really is, what depicted in the Ardhanarishvara. Some people, however, consider Siva as equal and inseparable aspect of Devi (Shakti), one can never be sure which concept really led to the creation (or whether was there really any concept to start with the sculpturing—we shall examine later) of the Ardhanarishvara. Ultimately of course the final conclusion reached is that Shakti and Shiva (Shaktiman—the masculine) are one and the same.[7] Each and every God in Hinduism has its partner or consort (here Shakti) and without this Shakti (consort), he is sometimes viewed as being without essential power. It is common practice to worship not just one personality but to combine it with its consort while worshipping. Traditionally, Krishna is often worshipped along with his consort Radha. Krishna is a childhood form of Vishnu. Krishna, as worshipped as "*bhagavan*", who is male, includes preference and veneration to his Radha (the female), who is worshipped as supreme. The union of Radha and Krishna may symbolize the union of Shakti with the Shaktiman. In Vaishnavism (a sect of Hinduism), Krishna is believed to be the source of all manifestations of God. Radha, his divine consort, is the original source of Shakti as feminine manifestation of divine force of energy.

In modern time, it is often said "behind every successful man, there is always a woman"—the woman is conceived as the source of driving force, the inspiration.

This concept is quite close to the Hindu concept of calling wife—*Ardhangini* (the half of body or better still the "better half"). This concept primarily highlights that the woman is an equal part of the man and vice versa. The Sanskrit marriage vow "Let my soul be thy and thy soul mine" clearly states the unification of two souls.

It is this concept, in the eye of a modern age man, is what is depicted in the deity Ardhanarishvara.

Before leaving this section, let me clarify one concept. I have earlier commented rather loosely on unification of two forces in the deity Ardhanarishvara. Force should not be equated with energy. Energies cannot be combined. Several scientists starting with Einstein had attempted it theoretically, but they all failed. What the deity really represents in physical scientific term is the unification of energy (Shakti) with its originator (Shiva) or the other way. Matter and energy are interconvertible as shown by Einstein (Energy = Mass × Velocity^2). In physical scientific term (also in a philosophical sense), God is a vast source of energy where from matter (universe and life for example) originates and where matter (life) ends. That is the fundamental concept of Hindu philosophy.

Concept of Duality in Buddhism

During a recent visit to Bhutan, in the capital city of Thimphu, the author came across a painted sculpture of Lord Buddha, the top half of which was depicted as a male form and the bottom half as a female form **(Fig. 4)**.

This image of the Supreme Lord is supposed to highlight the concept of duality in the Buddhist religion. Dualism in Buddhism generally means the division between subject and object, which is an illusion. You are not in your head with the world outside, everything is interconnected and interdependent. This is because that is, that is because this is. With nondual awareness this insight is realized directly. In simple terms it means the union of two opposites; the self and the outside world; the body and the mind; and the good and the evil. This concept may be a little different from the religious philosophy associated with the creation of Ardhnarishwar—the union of Shiva and Parvati. However, it may be closer to the Vedantic philosophy of considering every human being as a part of the Supreme Lord as preached by Sri Ramakrishna and Swami Vivekananda.

THE CONCEPT OF ARDHANARISHVARA IN SCIENTIFIC MYSTICISM

Mysticism can be equated with religious philosophy as discussed in the preceding section. The basic concept expressed in the deity Ardhanari is the unification

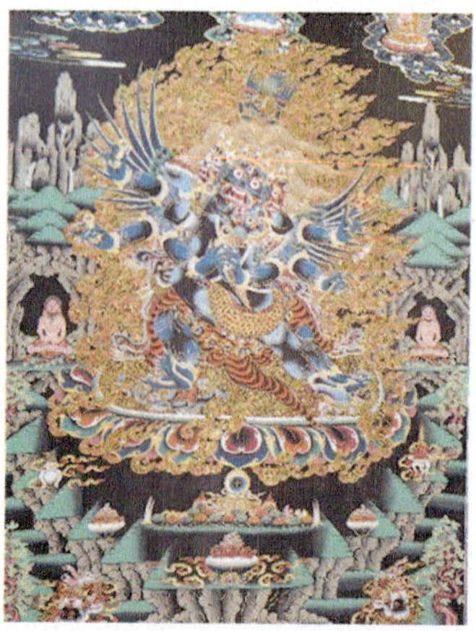

FIG. 4: Image of Lord Buddha depicting Duality.

of two opposites—the male Shiva and female Shakti. One of the fundamental principles of modern physics is that opposites unite at higher dimensions. As we talk about God as a vast conglomeration of energy, we refer to a multidimensional concept of a much higher order than what is now conceivable in Science (the four dimensions of Einstein's relativity).

The Austrian born American atomic physicist, Fritjof Capra, had written extensively on the parallels between modern physics and eastern mysticism especially in his best-selling book "The Tao of Physics".[8] Capra made a trip to Elephanta and marveled at the "Shiva Ardhanari", the stunning unification of male and female forms in the rhythmic, swaying movement of the deity's androgynous body. He referred this in his book—"Uncommon Wisdom".[9] He made brief note of Ardhanari in "The Tao of Physics" as well and a photograph of the Elephanta deity is included in the book.

Capra writes[8] "The most important characteristic of the Eastern World view—one could almost say the essence of it—is the awareness of the unity and mutual interrelation of all things and events, the experience of all phenomenon in the world as manifestations of a basic oneness". All things are seen as interdependent and inseparable parts of this cosmic whole, as different manifestation of the same ultimate reality. The Eastern traditions constantly refer to this ultimate, indivisible reality which manifests itself in all things, and of which all things are parts. As discussed earlier, Shakti is a part of Shiva and Shiva itself a part of Shakti. This oneness or unifying concept is what Hindus refer as Brahman, Buddhists refer as Dharmakaya, and Chinese as Tao. Fundamentally, in these concepts (or one concept), all differences and contrasts are relative within an all-embracing unity.

Capra brings in the conceptualizing "beyond the World of opposites"[8,9] to find the parallels between the eastern religious concept (mysticism) and modern physical concepts. Opposites are abstract concepts belonging to the realism of thought and as such they are relative. By the very act of focusing our attention on any one concept, we create its opposite. Good and bad, pleasure and pain, light and dark, and life and death are not absolute experiences belonging to different categories, but are two sides of the same reality—two poles which are set in a dynamic balance **(Fig. 5)**. Capra brings in the concept of "Yin" and "Yang" to explain the two poles beyond which lie the oneness, i.e., Tao.[8]

One of the principle polarities in life is the one between the male and female sides of human nature—and we usually bring one or the other side into

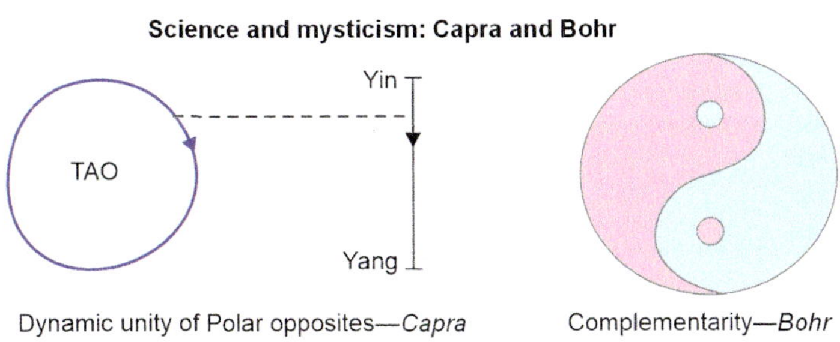

FIG. 5: The concept of Tao—dynamic unity of polar opposites and the concept of complementarity proposed by Niels Bohr.

prominence irrespective of the anatomical differences that exist between the two force. Capra felt that a unity between these two aspects of human nature is sought in Eastern mysticism. In support, he cites the example of the Ardhanari and the three-faced sculpture of Shiva Maheshwara, both seen at the Elephanta cave. He writes "... such a union of one's male and female modes can only be experienced on a higher plain of consciousness where the realm of thought and language is transcended and all opposites appear as a dynamic unity".[8] Just like as what had been said earlier relating to modern physics, opposites unite at higher dimensions.

Examples of the unification of opposite concepts in modern physics can be found at the subatomic level, where particles are both destructible and indestructible; where matter is both continuous and discontinuous and force and matter are but different aspects of the same phenomenon.

Space and time are two concepts which seemed entirely different but have been unified in relativistic physics. This fundamental unity is the basis of the unification of the opposite concepts. This unification, however, is only possible at a "higher plane" which is of higher dimensions.

It had taken physicists a long time to conceive the fact that matter manifests itself in ways which seem to be mutually exclusive and hence opposites. The prevailing concept, however, is that particles are waves and waves are also particles. Light, for example, is emitted and absorbed in the form of "quanta" or photons (particles) but when these particles of light travel through space, they appear as vibrating electric and magnetic fields which show all the characteristic behavior of waves. Likewise, electrons are normally considered to be particles and yet when a beam of these particles is sent through a small slit, it is diffracted just like a beam of light—particles behaving like a wave. Force and matter, particles and waves, and matter and rest—these are some of the opposite of contradictory concepts which are transcended in modern physics.

These various pairs of opposites can be conceptualized in the notion of complementarity. Capra[8,9] considered the particle picture and the wave picture as two complimentary description of the same reality. Bohr realized that the concept of complementarity can be a useful concept even outside the domain of physics and was impressed by the complementary concept in ancient China with the "Yin" and "Yang" lying at two opposite poles and complimentary to each other in Taoism. Similarly, Shakti and Shiva are complementary to each other in the deity Ardhanarishvara.

ARDHANARISHVARA: IN THE LIGHT OF NEUROSCIENCE

Having been trained as a clinical neurologist from an early age (and a thinking neurologist as trained by my mentors), I have developed a "bad" way of looking at most things from a neurological or neuroscientific perspective. As I often gazed at the small bronze replica of the Chola Ardhanari in my collection, I often wondered about the neuroscientific principle encoded in the sculpture. One day, rather suddenly, I had a vision which I would like to explain in this section. I shall explain my concept from the neurocognitive perspective first and then from the perspective of visual science (which of course is a sub-discipline of cognitive neuroscience).

I likened the two halves of the deity to the two halves of our brain—the left brain and the right brain. The left brain subserves language function, motor control of skilled movements, categorical processing, and arithmetic calculations. The right brain, on the other hand, houses function of spatial cognition, spatial imagery, face and object recognition, coordinative coding, and emotional communication. Looking differently, the left brain seems to have male characteristics (outspokenness, activity, rational thinking, competition, aggressiveness, and so on) whereas the right brain seems to harbor female characters like artistic talent, literary talent, religiousness, and love for the occult. Interestingly, the left half of Ardhanari is male form and right half depicts a female form—and they are united in the sculpture. This is exactly what is there in the human brain. The right brain and the left brain do not function independently but function as a whole in a most harmonious manner. This is because the two halves are united together by a thick bundle of white fibers called the corpus callosum. Every brain area of the left side is connected to corresponding area of the right and vice versa, although the areas might be responsible for different functions. Sectioning the corpus callosum (as may be needed for control of intractable epileptic seizures) lowers a person's creativity or novel ideation which is very closely dependent upon connectivity of brain circuits. Creative people always need the harmonious functioning of both halves of the brain in unison. Works of scientific or artistic creativity often require that one uses the skill and knowledge mediated by both halves of the brain. For example, the novelist who is writing about an emotional response of a character must use knowledge of facial emotional expression stored in the right brain together with the verbal lexicon stored in the left brain. The sculptor must imagine the rotation of spatial image mediated by the right brain while he uses the motor skill mediated by the left brain. The space physicist must combine the spatial computations mediated by the right brain with arithmetic skills mediated by the left brain.

We can thus appreciate how in neuroscience there is unity of two opposites—the right (female) brain and left brain (male). This is exactly what has been transpired in theories of modern physics—opposites unite at higher dimensions and brain's computing and thinking power is indeed multidimensional and beyond the range of any mathematical formulation. And interestingly, this is what is depicted in the Ardhanarishvara sculpture—the fusion of the opposites—Shiva and Shakti or simply a male and a female form.

My thought process in visual science in relation to Ardhanari is likely to raise controversy and criticism. While I do not wish to hurt the religious sentiment of any one but I need to give vent to my scientific reasoning. I am a devout Hindu who often practices idol worshipping, but still I cannot rise above the feeling of the scientist within.

I have a faint hesitation in accepting the fact, that the first artisan, who sculptured Ardhanarishvara, did so in the spirit of creating a Hindu deity. We assume that the earliest sculpture, dates to the early time of Kushana dynasty which reigned northern and central India. Now, the early Kushanas were not Hindus, they were, as stated earlier Buddhists with some western influence, depicted in their dresses and art forms. It is unlikely, therefore, that they would have patronized sculpturing a Hindu deity. Secondly, looking at least at the Elephanta sculpture (and Elephanta was probably not included within the Kushana empire as the historical maps suggest) and the Chola bronzes, it is apparent that the sculpture is essentially feminine. In fact, the female gender is inscribed in the very name—Ardhanari—a half female form. So my hypothesis is that originally the sculpture was crafted to depict just a beautiful sensuous female form. So what went wrong that the left half looks much like a male—the conspicuous thing being that the beautifully curved breast on the right chest is missing in the left. I tend to explain this by the phenomenon of hemineglect in the artisan who first crafted the original sculpture.

Hemineglect is a curious phenomenon in neuroscience where due to a lesion in one half of the brain (usually the right) caused commonly by a stroke, a person develops a "neglect" or unawareness in the opposite (i.e., the left) half of the field of vision. This is commonly tested by asking such a person to draw a clock face. A subject with a left hemineglect would miss out the numbers on the left half (viewer's or the subject's) of the clock face and would tend to put all or most of the numbers (from 1 to 12) on the right side (viewer's right) of the clock face. If such a subject happens to be an artist, this would be evident in the left half of his artwork which would be asymmetrical compared to the right or some features may be missing. Such phenomena had been recorded in a number of celebrated European artists including the famous German painter Lovis Corinth, following right brain stroke.[10] The artworks referred here include both painting and sculpture. The extent of the disability and hence the degree of distortion in the artwork depend on the degree of recovery of function after a brain injury (i.e., a stroke). I hypothesize that the original artisan who sculptured the Ardhanari suffered from left visual hemineglect due most probably from a right brain stroke. This explains the missing breast on the left half of the sculpture giving it a male form. And since it was a right brain injury, it did not affect his sculpturing skill (which rests in the left brain) and the right half had been crafted so beautifully. This phenomenon in the Ardhanarishvara is very similar to one of drawings available in a case of subarachnoid hemorrhage described by Lythgoe et al. clearly demonstrating left visual hemineglect **(Fig. 6)**.[11] I have a strong suspicion that the religious implications of the sculpture were conceptualized by later observers who were aware of the Hindu philosophical principles which were written in the Vedas much before the Kushana period.

CONCLUDING REMARKS

The final question is how does one feel when he or she stands in front the Elephanta sculpture or the Chola bronze. Does one think of religious philosophy or scientific mysticism or hard principles of neuroscience? One's vision and thoughts get flooded by the sheer beauty of the swaying androgynous sculpture. And beauty is the very essence of a creative artwork. Beauty elevates human subjectivity and human values to a transcendent level. A good piece of art, visual or otherwise, is a symbol of beauty and lies not in the eyes of the beholder but in his/her brain.

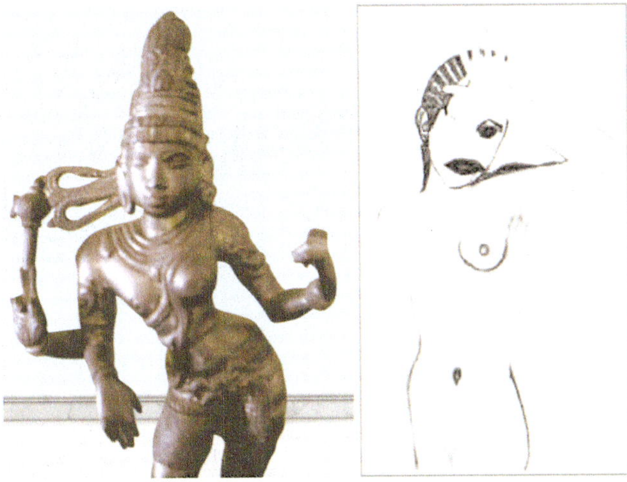

FIG. 6: Left visual hemineglect in Ardhanarishvara. Ardhanarishvara compared with a drawing of a female by an artist with left visual hemineglect.[11]

ACKNOWLEDGMENT

I wish to thank Late Professor AN Chakravarti of the Department of Radiophysics and Electronics, University College of Science, Calcutta and my wife Late Dr (Mrs) Srilekha Chakravarty for their help in the preparation of this manuscript.

REFERENCES

1. Kumar J. Masterpieces of Mathura Museum. New Delhi: Sundeep Prakashans; 2002.
2. Wikipedia. [online] Available from http://www.wikipedia.org [Last accessed February, 2025].
3. Shaivam.org. [online] Available from http://www.shaivam.org [Last accessed February, 2025].
4. Dvaita. [online] Available from http://www.dvaita.org [Last accessed February, 2025].
5. Bhattacharyya NN. History of Shakti religion. Delhi: Munsiram Monoharlal Publishers Ltd.; 1996.
6. Adishakti. [online] Available from http://www.adishakti.org [Last accessed February, 2025].
7. Kalkinath. Ardhanarishvara – the God who is half woman. [online] Available from http://www.philhine.org.uk [Last accessed February, 2025].
8. Capra F. The Tao of Physics. London: Flamingo; 1982.
9. Capra F. Uncommon Wisdom. London: Flamingo; 1989.
10. Bazner H, Hennerici MG. Painting after right hemisphere stroke case studies of professional artists. In: Bogousslavsky J, Hennerici MG (Eds). Neurological Disorders of Famous Artists. Basel: Karger; 2007. pp. 1-13.
11. Lythgoe MF, Pollak TA, Kalmus M, De Haan M, Chong WK. Obsessive, prolific artistic following subarachnoid hemorrhage. Neurology. 2005;64:397-8.

(Reprinted with modifications from Author's previous publication in Bulletin of Institute of Culture, Kolkata, India.)

INDEX

Page numbers followed by *f* refer to figure.

P

Q

R

S